Thread Lift in
Dermatology

Thread Lift in Dermatology

Editors

Indu Ballani MD
Consultant Dermatologist
Department of Dermatology
BLK-Max Super Speciality Hospital
New Delhi, India

Rashmi Sarkar MD(PGI) FAMS IFAAD
Director–Professor
Department of Dermatology
Lady Hardinge Medical College
New Delhi, India

JAYPEE
JAYPEE BROTHERS MEDICAL PUBLISHERS
The Health Sciences Publisher
New Delhi | London

JAYPEE **Jaypee Brothers Medical Publishers (P) Ltd**

Headquarters
EMCA House
23/23-B, Ansari Road, Daryaganj
New Delhi 110 002, India
Landline: +91-11-23272143, +91-11-23272703
+91-11-23282021, +91-11-23245672
E-mail: jaypee@jaypeebrothers.com

Overseas Office
J.P. Medical Ltd.
83, Victoria Street, London
SW1H 0HW (UK)
Phone: +44-20 3170 8910
E-mail: info@jpmedpub.com

Corporate Office
4838/24, Ansari Road, Daryaganj
New Delhi 110 002, India
Phone: +91-11-43574357
Fax: +91-11-43574314
E-mail: jaypee@jaypeebrothers.com

EU GPSR Authorised Representative
Logos Europe, 9 rue Nicolas Poussin
17000, La Rochelle, France
Phone: +33 (0) 6 67 93 73 78
E-mail: contact@logoseurope.eu

Website: www.jaypeebrothers.com
Website: www.jaypeedigital.com

Inquiries for bulk sales may be solicited at: jaypee@jaypeebrothers.com

Thread Lift in Dermatology / ***Indu Ballani, Rashmi Sarkar***

First Edition: 2025
Reprint: **2026**

ISBN: 978-93-6616-976-7

Printed in India

Dedication

This book is dedicated to

My family, whose unwavering love, support, and encouragement have been my greatest source of strength and inspiration.

My patients, who trust me with their care and continuously motivate me to learn, grow, and innovate.

The aesthetic dermatology community, for fostering an environment of collaboration and shared knowledge.

And to every practitioner who strives for excellence, this book is for you—may it guide and inspire you in your journey to mastering thread lifts.

With heartfelt gratitude!

Indu Ballani

This book is dedicated to my late parents,
Dr AK Sarkar and Mrs Chhobi Sarkar, my constant guiding force.

My family, who are my pillars of support.

My dear students and mentees, who have made the journey of teaching and learning rewarding.

The Almighty, who has always given fresh opportunities.

Rashmi Sarkar

Contributors

Aishwarya Raheja MBBS MD(Gold Medalist) DNB(Dermatology)
Consultant
Department of Dermatology
PN Behl Skin Institute
Greater Kailash, New Delhi, India

Damini Verma MBBS MD(Dermatology) DNB
Associate Consultant
Department of Dermatology
Apollomedics Hospital
Lucknow, Uttar Pradesh, India

Divya Asnani MD(Dermatology)
Senior Resident
Department of Dermatology
Dr DY Patil Medical College, Hospital and Research Centre
Pune, Maharashtra, India

Indu Ballani MD
Consultant Dermatologist
Department of Dermatology
BLK-Max Super Speciality Hospital
New Delhi, India

Rashmi Sarkar MD(PGI) FAMS IFAAD
Director–Professor
Department of Dermatology
Lady Hardinge Medical College
New Delhi, India

Preface

Writing this book has been a journey of learning, reflection, and collaboration, and I am deeply grateful to everyone who made it possible.

First and foremost, I extend my heartfelt thanks to my co-editor, Dr Rashmi Sarkar, for her unwavering support, meticulous guidance, and invaluable contributions. Her expertise and dedication have enriched this book in every way, making it a comprehensive resource for practitioners.

I am profoundly grateful to my family for their patience, encouragement, and love. Your belief in me has been my greatest strength throughout this endeavor.

A special thanks to the Aesthetic Zone Company for organizing thread training programs that allowed me to refine my skills and gain practical insights. These sessions not only deepened my knowledge but also gave me the confidence to share my methods with others.

This book was inspired by a conversation with a fellow dermatologist at a conference, who expressed the need for more accessible and practical literature on thread lifts. That moment sparked the idea of compiling my experiences and techniques into this book, and I hope it serves as a valuable guide for practitioners worldwide.

To every patient, colleague, mentor, and my juniors who have contributed to this book and my journey in aesthetics, thank you for shaping the knowledge and passion I bring to this field.

With gratitude!

Indu Ballani

Preface

Like every other event in the world, learning and education needs to evolve with time. Today dermatology is a vast subject with "Aesthetic Dermatology" occupying an important position. Learning has also increased in this sphere. As a Professor in Dermatology, I have always felt that besides studying for the curriculum, postgraduate students in Dermatology need to be future ready for their years in practice. So, I was happy when Dr Indu Ballani, an expert in "Aesthetic Dermatology" and a dear colleague, came to me with the idea of editing this little book with many of her tips. There are not really any books on this subject in this speciality.

I hope that this book is able to help those of our dermatologists who would like to practice the science of thread lifting methodically. Hope the readers find this little book interesting.

Warm regards!

Rashmi Sarkar

Contents

CHAPTER 1

History of Threads

Rashmi Sarkar, Aishwarya Raheja

INTRODUCTION

The origins of thread technology in medicine trace back to the 1960s when nonabsorbable threads were initially used for different surgical applications. These threads were made from materials that did not dissolve or break down in the body. The primary purpose of these threads was to provide mechanical support for tissues and organs, ensuring proper healing and alignment.

1960s—THE INCEPTION: NONABSORBABLE THREADS USED INITIALLY

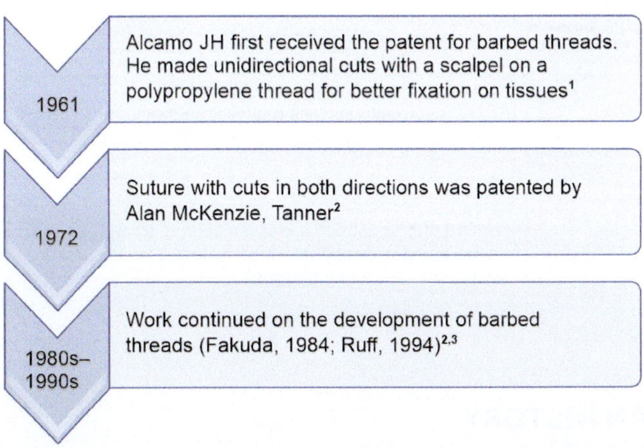

1990s—INTRODUCTION OF BIOABSORBABLE MATERIAL

The 1990s introduced a major shift in thread technology with the advent of bioabsorbable materials. This innovation allowed threads to gradually dissolve in the body over time, eliminating the need for removal. In 1999, MA Sulamanidze pioneered the use of Aptos Lift sutures, which were polypropylene threads with notches designed for tissue lifting. His research, published in 2000, demonstrated the efficacy of these threads in nonsurgical facial lifting procedures.

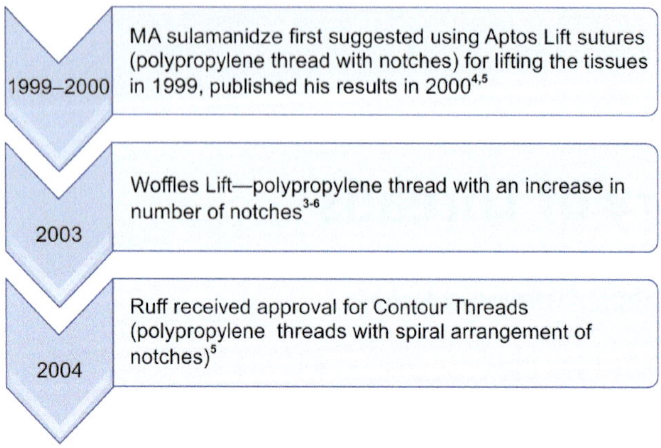

2000s—FOOD AND DRUGS ADMINISTRATION APPROVAL AND EVOLUTION OF THREADS

The early 2000s saw further advancements in thread technology. This design provided enhanced lifting effects and contributed to the growing popularity of thread-based procedures. Additionally, ISSE proposed using polypropylene threads with resorbable cones (Silhouette Lift) as an alternative to notches.

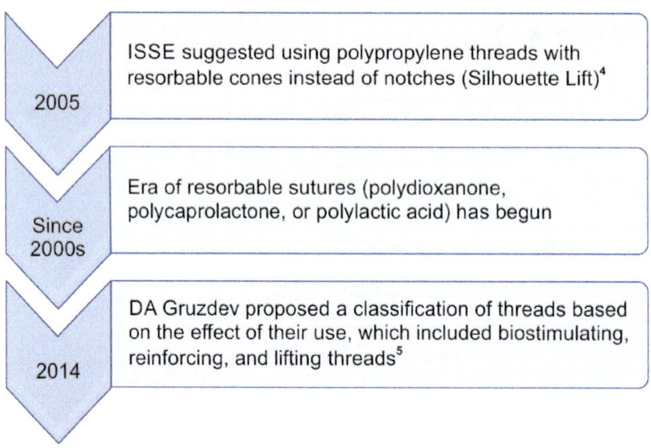

INDIAN HISTORY

India saw significant developments in thread technology between 2012 and 2021. In 2012, Aakar introduced mono threads, which were biocompatible, biodegradable, and made from polydioxanone (PDO). This innovation marked a significant step forward in the Indian market. Medizone aesthetics followed with the introduction of mono screw/twin screw threads for skin rejuvenation and broom threads for nasolabial folds in 2013. In 2014, Alfa Aqulift brought cog threads to India, featuring conventional cutting barbs on a PDO base.

The introduction of silhouette thread lift in 2015, also known as the "lunchtime facelift," used specialized poly L-lactic acid (PLLA) bioabsorbable sutures with resorbable bidirectional cones. By 2016, TESSLIFT SOFT, a 3D mesh scaffold made from PDO material, was introduced. The MINT™ (Minimally Invasive Nonsurgical Thread) system, launched in 2018, became notable for being the first PDO threads with triple FDA clearances. In 2021, Aptos, featuring multidirectional absorbable threads composed of Poly Lactic acid/Caprolactone, and Definisse threads/Happy Lift™ threads, which combined immediate lifting with prolonged revitalizing actions, were introduced in India.

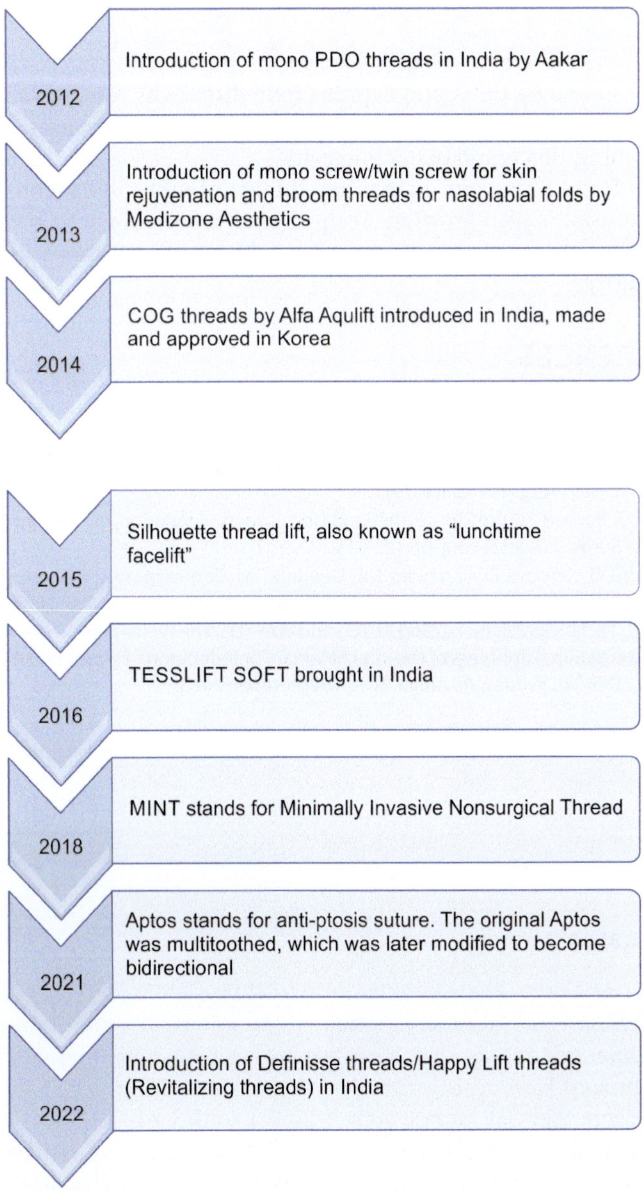

CLINICAL PEARL

Understanding the history of threads provides valuable insights into their evolution from early surgical sutures to modern day nonsurgical treatments.

CONCLUSION

In the modern era, nonsurgical face lift has become increasingly popular among patients seeking less invasive options for facial lifting. As a result of ongoing research and development, improvements are being made in material and insertion methods of threads.

Barbed threads are now being used for its better lifting effect. Today, PDO threads are joined by PLLA and caprolactone threads as research shows P(LA/CL) threads induce more collagen formation and tissue responses, resulting in more tightening effects and better longevity.

Besides facial lifting and tightening, the list of other indications for which threads are used is also growing. Scalp threads have shown to stimulate hair regrowth. Nose threads, eyebrow threads, and body threads have also begun to gain popularity.

REFERENCES

1. Alcamo JH. Surgeon's Suturing Device. US Patent 2,988,028. 1961.
2. Ruff GL. The history of barbed sutures. Aesthet Surg J. 2013;33(3 Suppl):12S-6S.
3. Wu WTL. Commentary on facial rejuvenation with fine barbed threads: The simple MIZ-lift. Aesthetic Plast Surg. 2014;38(1):75-7.
4. Paul MD. Barbed sutures in aesthetic plastic surgery: Evolution of thought and process. Aesthet Surg J. 2013;33(3 Suppl):17S-31S.
5. Borzykh OB, Karpova EI, Shnayder NA, Demina OM. Contemporary view on thread lifting: Histological and anatomical approaches. Russian Open Medical Journal. 2022;11:e0107.
6. Wu WTL. Facial rejuvenation using APTOS and WAPTOS (the Woffles lift): a novel approach. In: 13th International Congress of the International Confederation of Plastic and Reconstructive Surgery (IPRAS), Sydney, Australia, 10–14 September, 2003.

CHAPTER 2

Anatomy Relevant to Thread Lifting

Aishwarya Raheja, Divya Asnani

INTRODUCTION

Comprehension of anatomy is an important basis for a Dermatologist to deliver the best results for a successful and effective thread lift. A thorough understanding of the underlying structures of the face and neck, including muscles, fat pads, and connective tissues, enables dermatologists to make informed decisions about placement and technique. Additionally, it is essential to recognize that the skin can vary significantly based on factors such as gender, age, and ethnicity, which can influence the overall outcome of the treatment. Each patient presents unique anatomical features that require a tailored approach. By integrating anatomical knowledge with an awareness of individual characteristics, we can optimize results, enhance patient satisfaction, and minimize complications, ensuring a safe and effective thread-lifting experience.

Basic facial soft tissues are composed of five layers **(Fig. 1)**:[1]

1. Skin
2. Subcutaneous layer
3. Superficial musculoaponeurotic system (SMAS)
4. Retaining ligament and spaces
5. Periosteum and deep fascia

THICKNESS OF THE SKIN

Epidermis in Indians is thicker than Caucasians. The general thickness of the skin varies at different sites. The skin layer of the anterior cheek and the mental region are relatively thicker when compared to upper and lower eyelids, glabella, and nasal region, which have an exceptionally thin skin.[2] Males have a thicker skin than females. However, thickness of dermis is almost same in both.

SUPERFICIAL SUBCUTANEOUS FAT

This layer corresponds to the hypodermis. The subcutaneous fat tissue of the face tends to sag due to gravity. It is divided into various compartments as described here **(Fig. 2)**:[3]

- *Forehead fat*:
  - Central forehead compartment
  - Middle forehead compartment
- *Orbital fat*:
  - Superior orbital fat
  - Inferior orbital fat

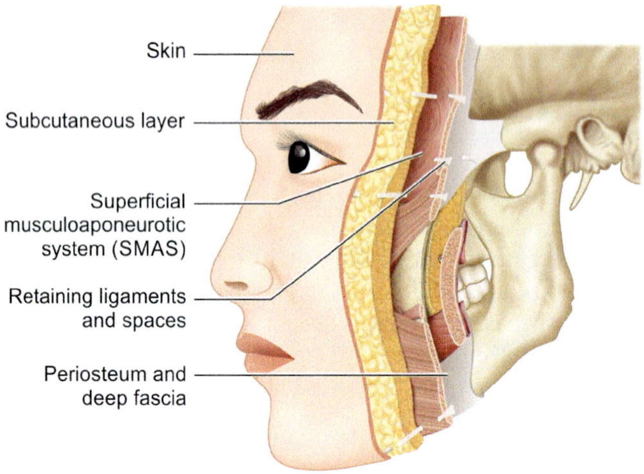

FIG. 1: Facial layers.

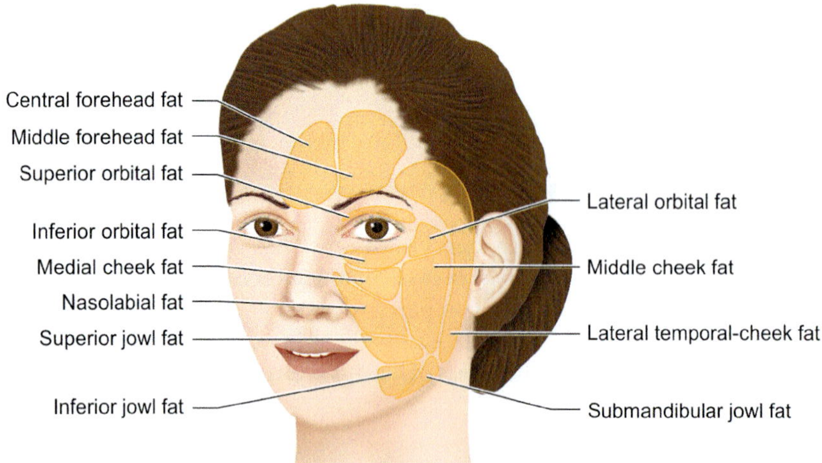

FIG. 2: Superficial fat compartments.

- *Lateral facial fat*:
  - Lateral temporal fat
  - Lateral orbital fat
  - Lateral cheek fat
- *Malar fat*:
  - Superficial infraorbital fat compartment
  - Nasolabial fat compartment
  - Medial cheek fat compartment
- *Jowl fat*:
  - Superior jowl fat
  - Inferior jowl fat
- *Mental fat*: However, the boundary is not visible to the naked eye.

SUPERFICIAL MUSCULOAPONEUROTIC SYSTEM

The SMAS is a continuous and organized network of fibrotic septa that connects the facial muscles to dermis. It extends from the platysma to the galea aponeurotic and is continuous with the superficial temporal fascia and the galea layer.[4]

It constitutes three distinct layers; a fascial layer superficial to the muscles, a layer closely associated with the facial muscles, and a deep layer attached to the periosteum of facial bones.

DEEP FAT AND RETAINING LIGAMENTS

There are several important deep fat pads and retaining ligaments in the fourth layer of face.[5] Deep fat pad is located deep to the facial expression muscles and are divided into several compartments described below **(Fig. 3)**:

- *Orbital fat*: The SOOF (suborbicularis oculi fat) covers the zygomatic bone and creates a gliding pad for the malar eminence soft tissue. The ROOF

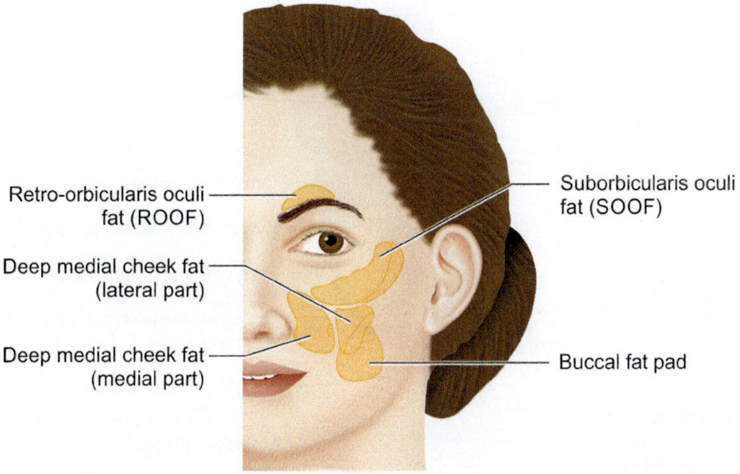

FIG. 3: Deep fat compartments.

(retro-orbicularis oculi fat) covers the lateral part of the supraorbital rim and creates a cushion for the eyebrow.

- *Deep medial cheek fat*: It is quite a large compartment with great cosmetic relevance as its volume decreases with age, affecting the facial shape. The zygomaticus major muscle forms its lateral surface, and zygomaticocutaneous ligament forms the upper border. It is located underneath the lip elevator muscles and in the infraorbital space. It is divided into medial and lateral parts by the lateral border of the levator angular oris muscle or the facial veins.
- *Buccal fat*: This fat compartment envelops the coronoid process and the temporalis tendon. It also has a buccal extension protruding just anterior to the masseter muscle.
- *Deep mental fat*: The deep mental fat pad covers the mental protuberance under the mentalis muscle. It acts as a gliding pad for the mental soft tissue.

CUTANEOUS RETAINING LIGAMENTS

The face has several retaining ligaments that firmly support the soft tissue **(Fig. 4)**. These ligaments can be broadly divided on the basis of their strength, attachment, and function into:

- *True (osteocutaneous) ligaments*: The true retaining ligament arises from the periosteum and attaches to the dermis. The zygomatic ligament, lateral orbital thickening ligament, and the mandibular ligament are the examples of true retaining ligaments.
- *False (fasciocutaneous) ligaments*: The false retaining ligament originates from the dermis and attaches to the underlying SMAS. The orbicularis retaining ligament, zygomatic cutaneous ligament, and masseteric cutaneous ligament are the examples of false retaining ligaments.

The ligaments are particularly strong over the forehead, eyes, nose, lip, and chin; of intermediate strength over the medial cheek and temple areas and

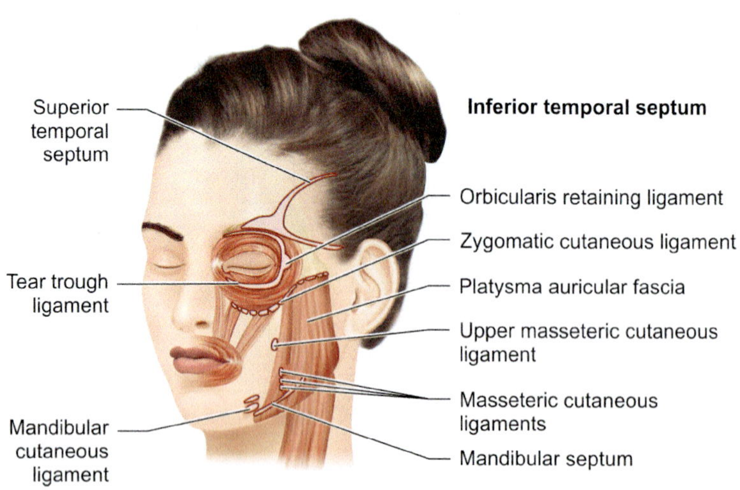

FIG. 4: Cutaneous retaining ligaments.

relatively loose over medial cheek and temple areas. As a result, these ligaments easily lose elasticity and sag with age, causing fat redistribution and sagging.

CLINICAL PEARL

- Selecting the right vectors that target these ligaments, helps in facial contouring similar to tent being pulled by tight ropes.
- Therefore, threads not only play an important role in superficial fat pad repositioning but an overall contouring.
- Combination treatments may be required when deep fat pads get involved.

ANATOMICAL RISK ZONES

Although thread lifting is a minimally invasive procedure, there is a risk of injury to structures, which run horizontally or obliquely in the lateral face.

Blood Vessels

The risk of vascular complications relating to thread lifting is minimal when compared to the filler injection. However, chances of bleeding is comparatively higher while performing thread lifting that may present with bruising, hematoma, edema, and pain.[6]

Branches of superficial temporal artery, which are at risk, are summarized here **(Fig. 5)**:

- *Frontal branch*: It arises from superficial temporal artery around 18 mm anterior and 37 mm superior to tragus. It courses anterosuperiorly in the temple, meeting the lateral border of frontalis 15 mm above the eyebrow and 16 mm lateral to the lateral canthus.
- *Zygomatico-orbital artery*: It travels parallel to the upper border of zygomatic arch toward to the lateral canthus.

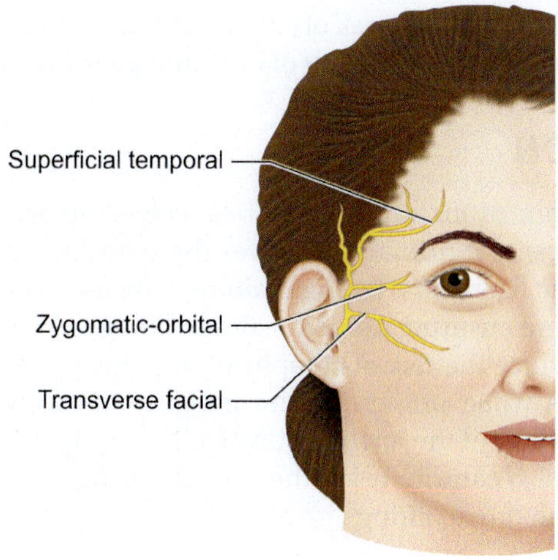

FIG. 5: Important arteries in thread lifting.

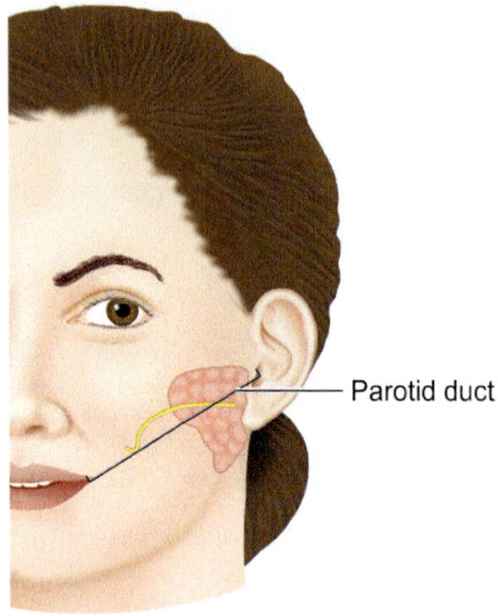

FIG. 6: The course of the parotid duct.

- *Transverse facial artery*: It arises within the parotid gland, courses in between the parotid gland and zygomatic arch (approximately 14 mm below the lower border of zygomatic arch).

  When thread passes through the parotid gland, make sure it stays in the subcutaneous layer to prevent injury to the transverse facial artery.
- *Middle temporal vein*: It runs between the superficial and deep layers of the deep temporal fascia, approximately 2 cm above the zygomatic arch.
- *Nerves*: The possibility of nerve damage is minimal if threads are inserted in the right plane. The zygomatic arch is the most likely place for damage to facial nerve as the thickness of the soft tissues is relatively thin at this area and facial nerve passes close to the bone.
- *Parotid duct*: It traverses above the line connecting the tragus and angle of mouth following a curved trajectory from the one-third point and two-thirds point along the line with the peak of curve being 1.5 cm above the line **(Fig. 6)**. The duct may be injured if our layer of insertion goes wrong.

CONCLUSION

The anatomy relevant to thread lifting is relatively simpler compared to other aesthetic procedures, as it primarily involves the repositioning of superficial fat pads toward specific ligaments. By maintaining a focused understanding of the anatomical layers and ensuring proper insertion along the designated tracks, we can significantly reduce the risk of complications. This precise approach allows for effective results while preserving the integrity of surrounding structures. Ultimately, a solid grasp of the anatomy involved not only enhances the safety of the procedure but also contributes to the overall satisfaction of patients seeking rejuvenation through thread lifting.

REFERENCES

1. Halepas S, Chen XJ, Ferneini EM. Thread-Lift Sutures: Anatomy, Technique, and Review of Current Literature. J Oral Maxillofac Surg. 2020;78(5):813-20.
2. Jeong KM, Seo JY, Kim A, Kim YC, Baek YS, Oh CH, et al. Ultrasonographic analysis of facial skin thickness in relation to age, site, sex, and body mass index. Skin Res Technol. 2023;29(8):e13426.
3. Zachary C, Grushchak S, Newman J. Skin Anatomy and Analysis. Facial Plast Surg Clin North Am. 2023;31(4):433-42.
4. Kim HJ, Seo KK, Lee HK, Kim J (Eds). Clinical Anatomy of the Face for Filler and Botulinum Toxin Injection. Singapore: Springer; 2016.
5. Kim B, Oh S, Jung W (Eds). The Art and Science of Thread Lifting. Singapore: Springer; 2019.
6. Daskalopoulou D, Matsas A, Chrysikos D, Troupis T. The Superficial Temporal Artery. Acta Med Acad. 2023;51(3):232-42.

CHAPTER 3

Types of Threads

Aishwarya Raheja

INTRODUCTION

Facial ageing is a cumulative result of gravity, bone absorption, fat redistribution, and decreased tissue elasticity. The use of threads in aesthetic medicine is gaining a lot of popularity because of its immediate lifting and revitalizing action. The mechanical properties of thread produce tissue repositioning and provides support to tissues. The biorevitalizing properties of threads stimulates synthesis of collagen, hyaluronic acid, and elastin.

Threads can be classified based on several standards, and selection of threads depends on the desired outcome.[1]

CLASSIFICATION OF THREADS

- *Based on material*: Nonabsorbable versus absorbable:
  - Nonabsorbable: They remain permanently in the subdermal tissue. They only have a lifting action. The examples are: Polypropylene/prolene, gold, and silicone
  - Absorbable: They have a limited lifetime as the enzymatic action hydrolyses them. Absorbable threads have both lifting and revitalizing action.[1]

    The examples are:
    - PDO (polydioxanone)
    - PCL (polycaprolactone)
    - PLLA (poly-L-lactic acid)

  Properties of different materials of absorbable threads are described in **Table 1**.[2,3]
- *Presence of cogs/cones*: Smooth/Nonsmooth
  - Nonsmooth threads have small projections (barbs or cones) that radiate outward from the center of the thread **(Fig. 1)**. The main purpose of these structural elements is anchorage and repositioning of soft tissues.

    The examples of barbed threads are: Definisse, APTOS, and Mintlift.

    The example of cones is: Silhouette soft[1]

TABLE 1: Comparison between different absorbable threads.

Features	PDO	PCL	PLLA
Collagen stimulation	Type 1	Type 1 and 3	Type 1
Biodegradation period	6–8 months	16–24 months	12–18 months
Flexibility	Average	High	Low
Discomfort	Moderate	Slight	Strong

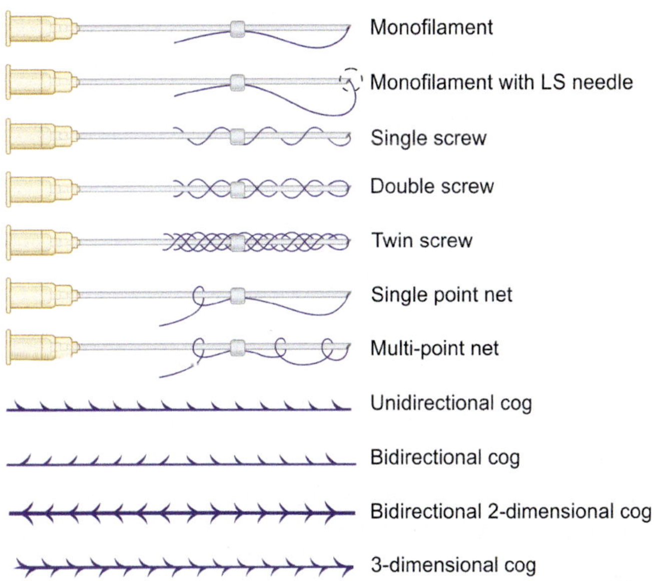

FIG. 1: Different types of absorbable threads.

- Smooth threads (nonbarbed) lack an anchoring mechanism and are mainly used for biorevitalization.

  The examples of smooth threads are: Mono threads and cog screw threads **(Fig. 1)**.
- *Direction of cog*: Unidirectional versus bidirectional **Flowchart 1**:
  - Unidirectional: All barbs are angled in one direction. The example is: Definisse anchorage threads.
  - Bidirectional (convergent/divergent): Barbs are present in opposite direction with a central smooth area to promote gripping and tissue accumulation in the middle of the thread.

    The examples of bidirectional convergent threads are Definisse free floating and double needle threads.

    The example of bidirectional divergent is Boca threads (Definisse).
  - Multidirectional: Barbs alternate directions throughout the whole thread.

    The example of multidirectional is: APTOS threads
- *Shape of needle*: Cannula type versus needle
- *Manufacturing method of cog*: Cutting versus molding

First generation of threads
- First to be introduced
- Example: Thin mono thread
- Only revitalizing action

↓

Second generation of threads
- Thread in a twister shape
- Better revitalizing action than mono threads

↓

Third generation of threads
- Cutting thread with cog
- Most of the Korean brands that were initially available were of cutting type
- Lifting + revitalizing action

↓

Fourth generation of threads
- Bidirectional molding cog
- Latest with maximum lifting and revitalizing action because of molding technology

FLOWCHART 1: Evolution of threads.

  - Molding is a manufacturing process that improves tensile strength of the threads. It involves simultaneously pressing the body and barbs of the thread.[1]
- *Twisting of thread*: Simple versus twister
- *Length of thread*: Long versus short

> CLINICAL PEARL
>
> Choosing the right product and the right vector is the key to achieve satisfactory outcome.

COMMON BRANDS AVAILABLE IN INDIA

- *APTOS*: APTOS stands for antiptosis suture. These are absorbable multi-directional threads composed of P(LA/CL) (poly-L-lactic acid and caprolactone). Their product line includes cog and double needle threads with or without hyaluronic acid.
- *MINT*: MINT stands for minimally invasive nonsurgical thread. MINT threads are made up of polydioxanone or PDO. These threads are made by using patented technology where the barbs are press-molded on the surface in a 360° helical pattern. These are the first and only PDO threads with triple FDA clearances **(Table 2)**.
- *Definisse*: Definisse threads/Happy Lift™ are a range of absorbable, monofilament, barbed threads of synthetic origin P(LA/CL).

  These threads interact with tissue in double action to provide the following benefits: Immediate lifting action, and prolonged revitalizing action stimulating collagen, hyaluronic acid, and elastin.

- *Definisse free floating threads*: These are bidirectional and convergent threads. These threads are indicated in cases where a good anteromedial projection is desired. The available lengths are 12 cm and 23 cm.
- *Definisse double needle threads*: These are also bidirectional and convergent threads. The thread ends with two straight triangular needles. These threads give a good jawline definition and lifting effect. The available lengths are 12 cm and 23 cm.
- *Definisse anchorage threads*: These are unidirectional barbed threads that lift the face by anchorage at the temples. It is only available in 12.6 cm. These are mostly used by plastic surgeons.

- *APHRODITE* **(Table 3)**:
  - Specialized in PDO, P(LA/CL), and PLLA
  - P(LA/CL) is an ideal product that overcomes weakness of PLLA and PCL with a powerful and long-lasting lifting performance **(Flowchart 2)**.

TABLE 2: Product line of MINT threads available in India.

Product line	Barb design	Thread length	Cannula type/ needle gauges	Indications
MINT FINE+	Bidirectional	18 cm	18G W cannula	Face
MINT PETIT+	Bidirectional	15 cm	19G W cannula	Eyebrow
MINT TIP	Bidirectional	4 cm	19G L cannula	Nose
MINT UP	Multidirectional	9.5 cm	19G L cannula	Nose
MINT MONO	Smooth, no barbs	3/5/7/9 cm	Needle gauges—25G/27G/29G/30G	Rejuvenation
MINT EASY	Bidirectional	43 cm	19G sharp needle	Double needle threads for better lifting

TABLE 3: Product line of APHRODITE threads available in India.

Product line	Barb design	Thread length	Cannula type/ needle gauze	Indications
SC molding	USP 1-0/2-0	185 mm	W-type cannula 18/19G	Face
FA nose	USP 1-0	80 mm	L-type cannula 21G	Nose
FG nose	USP 2-0	50 mm	L-type cannula 19G	Nose
Cavern screw	USP 5-0	25/30 mm	L-type cannula 23G	Jawline
Multi-fill	USP 5-0	25/45 mm	L-type cannula 23G	Nasolabial folds
Mono	Smooth/ Nonbarbed	60/80 mm	29G	Forehead, mid/lower face, double chin, neck, body parts

Continued

Continued

Product line	Barb design	Thread length	Cannula type/ needle gauze	Indications
Mono	Smooth/ Nonbarbed	30 mm	30G	Hair, crow's feet, lips, under eye wrinkles, perioral lines, Marionette lines
Screw	Smooth/ Nonbarbed	60/70 mm	27G	Forehead, mid/lower face, double chin, neck, body parts

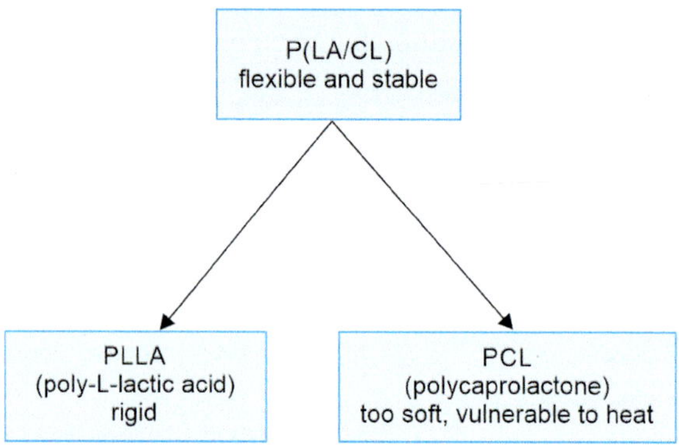

FLOWCHART 2: Aphrodite threads.

- All products are produced in Korea.
- The greatest quality secured by CE, GMP, and ISO.

- *Bio-meyisun threads*: The product line includes all varieties of PDO threads distributed by a Mumbai-based company "Medizone Aesthetics".
- *Aakar/Aqulift threads*: These threads are CE, TGA, GOST, IMVIMA, and COFEPRIS approved and made in Korea by Alfa medical.

Their product line includes cog threads, mono threads, and double screw threads. Only PDO threads are available in India.

CONCLUSION

Thread lift is the best option for those seeking nonsurgical face lift. Since this procedure has been gaining popularity, there has been a continuous influx of newer types of threads in the market. The latest ones include double needle, free floating and APTOS NAMICA threads (PLA encapsulation of hyaluronic acid which increases longevity of results). There has also been a shift from PDO to P(LA/CL) threads because of better longevity of P(LA/CL) threads.

REFERENCES

1. Kim B, Oh S, Jung W. Evolution of absorbable thread lifting. In: Oh SM, Hong G, Song W (Eds). The Art and Science of Thread Lifting. Singapore: Springer; 2019. pp. 65-7.
2. Wong V, Rafiq N, Kalyan R, Hsenriksen A, Funner R. Hanging by a thread: choosing the right thread for the right patient. J Dermat Cosmetol. 2017;1(4):86-8.
3. Cao L, Qiu H, Yu D, Shuo L, Wang H. Comparison of different thread products for facial rejuvenation: Materials and barb designs. J Cosmet Dermatol. 2023;22(7):1988-94.

CHAPTER 4

Patient Selection and Counseling

Indu Ballani

INTRODUCTION

Choosing an ideal candidate is the most important step toward achieving satisfactory outcome of a procedure. Although, this comes with experience but some points can be kept in mind before counseling a patient for threads.

PATIENT EVALUATION

Before recommending threads to your patients, it is essential to consider the following factors:

- *Age*: Thread lift generally gives better results in patients in their 30s to 60s who have mild-to-moderate sagging. Excessive sagging makes them a better surgical candidate.
- *Skin quality*: Thread lift would be more effective if patients have a relatively good skin quality with moderate to good skin thickness. Polycaprolactone (PCL) micro barbed threads like Definisse and Aptos can be used in patients with thin skin, although results may vary. Thicker barbed cog threads are more suitable for heavier faces.
- *Facial anatomy*: A good evaluation of the descended superficial fat pads, laxity of the ligaments, muscle tone, and deep fat pads is essential to plan the full treatment regimen. In cases where loss of volume is evident, especially in the deep fat pads (hypotrophic/ptotic), a combination treatment with fillers may be required.
- *Expectations*: While counseling the patients, it is important that we understand patient's expectations and set realistic goals for them.
- *Medical history*: Taking a detailed history regarding previous procedures, allergies, or medications is important to reduce the risk of complications.

IDEAL CANDIDATE

An ideal candidate has the following characteristics:

- Mild-to-moderated laxity on the cheeks, visibly descended jowls, neck laxity. If we try to lift the skin with our hands, we are able to lift more than 1–1.5 cm of the skin.
- Good overall health with no contraindications to the procedure
- Realistic expectations
- Willingness to follow pre- and postprocedure instructions
- No major social obligations for minimum 7–10 days after the procedure

COUNSELING PATIENTS

Some of the key points that should be kept in mind at the time of counseling are described here.

- *Explaining the procedure*: A detailed explanation of the type and number of threads, potential risks, areas to be covered, and expected recovery should be given.
- *Expected results*: Discuss the anticipated outcome by holding a mirror in front of them **(Fig. 1)**. Also, discuss the vectors which would benefit them. Do not over-pull with your hand at the time of counseling, to avoid giving unrealistic expectations.
- *Risks and complications*: A detailed information about all the risks involved that includes bruising, swelling, and infection, should be given and consent forms should be signed.

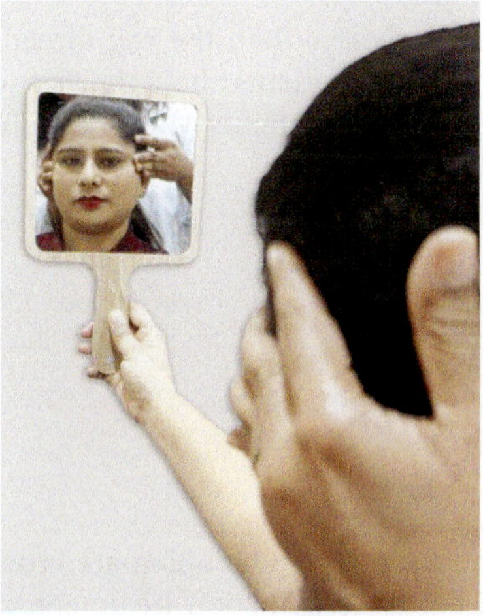

FIG. 1: Comparing the different vectors on both sides to choose a better vector for insertion.

- *Aftercare instructions*: It is necessary to discuss all the aftercare even before the procedure including any activity restriction and follow-up appointments.
- *Cost and financing*: Discussing the expenses is also an important aspect of the counseling as the patients should be made aware of the varying results, which can be achieved with different budgets depending on the type and number of threads they are choosing.

CHOOSING TYPE OF THREADS AND VECTORS

We have a wide range of threads available nowadays and choosing the best threads for a particular face-type according to their budget is sometimes a dilemma.[1]

Cog Threads

Cog threads are chosen when an instant lift is required with minimal entry and exit points. When the budget is less, polydioxanone (PDO) cog threads are usually chosen. Patients should be made aware that although PCL threads are more expensive but they have a better longevity.

Discussing vectors: Minimum eight cog threads are required to give a good lift. The results of various vectors should be explained to the patients by comparing the results on both sides. For example, patient's concern might be nasolabial folds but on comparing vectors on both sides, the temple vectors going down to the jowl might be giving better results if only four threads are being used, compared to the direct vectors for nasolabial folds.

Double Needle Threads (Definisse) or Aptos Threads

These threads are more expensive than the cog threads. Counseling for these threads includes explaining the patients about the finer quality of these threads. These threads are better suited in patients who have thinner skin and thinner fat pads where repositioning is required.

> **CLINICAL PEARL**
>
> Any face where we can lift 1 cm or more of skin, is good for a thread procedure but counseling is important so that the expectations are according to the amount of material being taken.

CONCLUSION

Thorough counseling and procedure planning are crucial for ensuring patient satisfaction. In several cases, combination treatment with fillers and toxins is required to achieve optimal aesthetic results.

REFERENCE

1. Wong V, Rafiq N, Kalyan R, Hsenriksen A, Funner R. Hanging by a thread: choosing the right thread for the right patient. J Dermat Cosmetol. 2017;1(04):86-8.

CHAPTER 5

Mono Threads: Uses and Insertion

Indu Ballani, Aishwarya Raheja

INTRODUCTION

Mono threads are the first-generation absorbable threads designed to tighten and rejuvenate the skin. Mono threads are made up of a material called polydioxanone (PDO), which stimulates type 1 collagen production, creating a tightening effect for almost 6–12 months.

Recently, mono threads made up of poly-L-lactic acid and caprolactone P(LA/CL) material have been launched in India. These threads stimulate both collagen 1 and 3 production with a longer lasting tightening effect.

USES OF MONO THREADS

- *Facial rejuvenation*: Mono threads are a novel, minimally invasive treatment option for promoting collagen production and smoothing the skin. Thus, improve the appearance of fine lines.
- *Lifting*: Mono threads can give a mild lift along with the skin boosting effect. The vectors for lifting with mono are described in **Figure 1**.

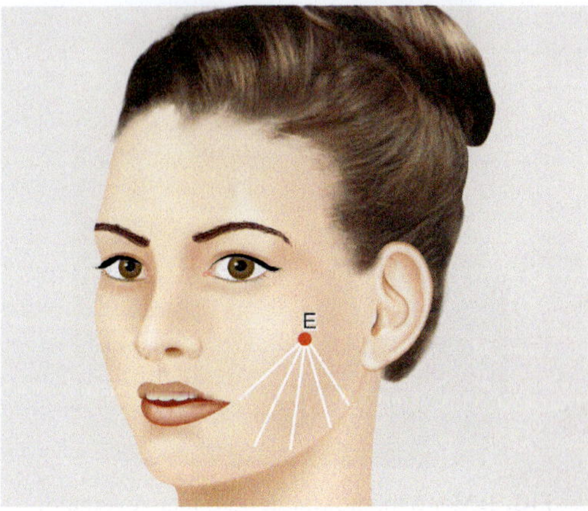

FIG. 1: Vectors for lifting with mono/cog screw threads.

- *Scar reduction*: It is postulated that absorbable threads promote tissue regeneration by fibroblast activation. Mono threads give promising results when used for atrophic acne scars.[1] Mono threads are inserted in a meshwork when the indication is scar reduction **(Fig. 2)**.
- *Periorbital rejuvenation*: Patients with mild-to-moderate wrinkling and textural changes in periorbital area reported higher degree of satisfaction with mono threads (PDO, 25 mm) compared to those with severe wrinkling and under eye bags **(Fig. 3)**.[2]
- *Scalp threads*: These are mono threads 12–25 mm in length. They improve hair density, thickness, and appearance. They are used in combination with minoxidil in androgenetic alopecia **(Fig. 4)**.[3,4]

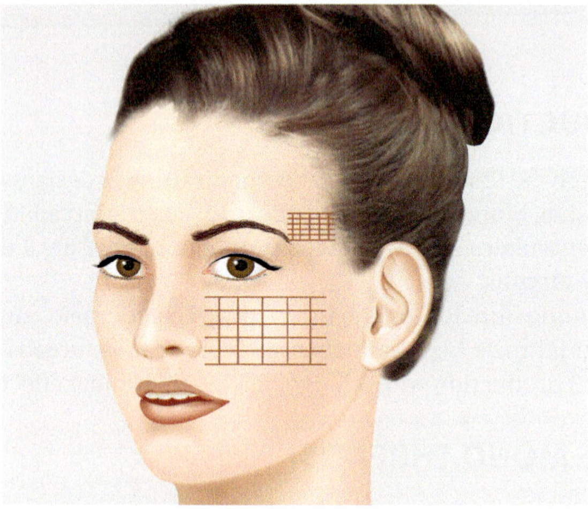

FIG. 2: Vectors for acne scars.

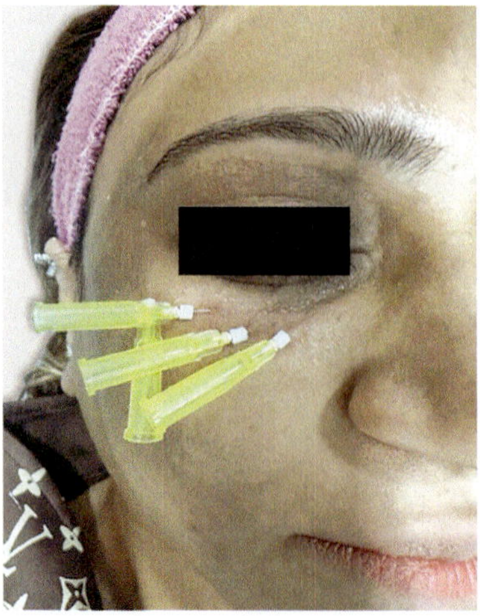

FIG. 3: Mono threads for periorbital rejuvenation.

- *Forehead rejuvenation*: Mono threads can also be used to improve textural appearance of the forehead, brow, and area around the eye.
- *Neck rejuvenation*: Mono threads can address the wrinkled, loose, inelastic, and sagged skin of neck by stimulating collagen production and neoangiogenesis.[5]
- *Body threads*: Mono threads are also used to improve the appearance of stretch marks and for abdominal tightening in combination with cog threads **(Fig. 5)**. They can be used on any part of the body where firming and tightening is required. For these indications, longer mono threads are used.[6]

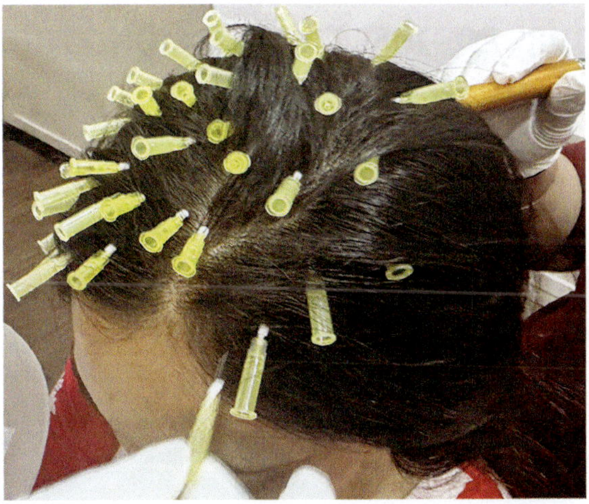

FIG. 4: Scalp threads in a case of female pattern hair loss.

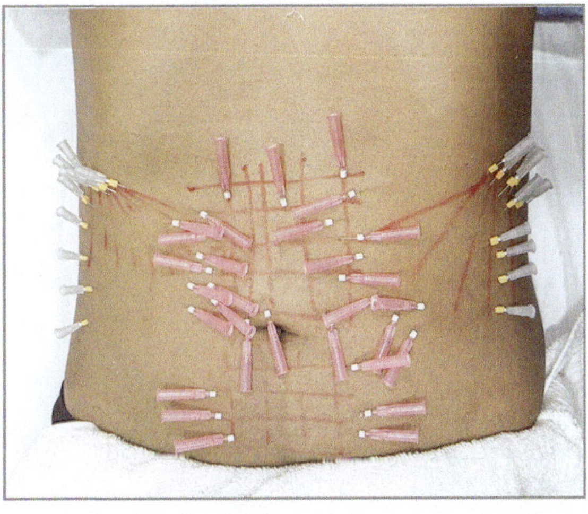

FIG. 5: Mono threads in combination with cog threads for abdominal tightening.

LENGTH OF MONO THREAD AND INDICATION

Table 1 shows the length of mono thread with indication.

THE VECTORS FOR MONO AND SCREW THREADS

Vectors do not matter for mono thread as they are smooth threads and can be inserted in any direction. When we are inserting for acne scars or in the cheek area we prefer mesh formation to rejuvenate the skin. When corkscrew threads are being used the may be inserted in a fan shaped pattern as shown in **Figure 1** from a common point of insertion.

PROCEDURE FOR INSERTION OF MONO THREADS

- Mark the vectors **(Figs. 1 and 6)**.
- Stretch the skin.
- Insert the thread in an oblique direction in deep dermal layer as in subcision **(Fig. 7)**.

TABLE 1: Types of mono threads and indications.

Length of mono thread	Indication
25 mm	Scalp, periorbital, and forehead
38 mm	Double chin, neck, and forehead
50 mm	Face and neck
70 mm	Body

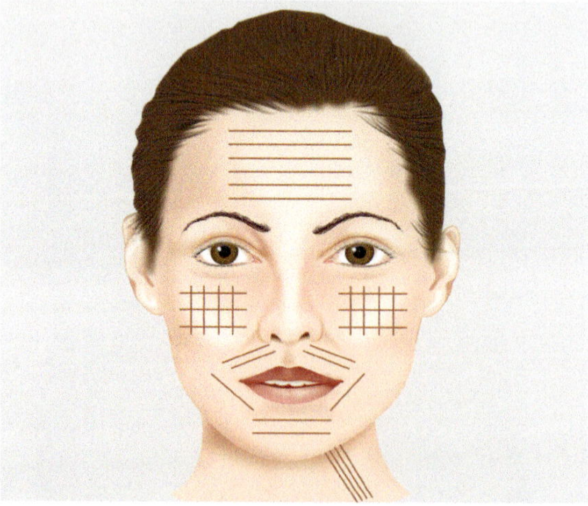

FIG. 6: Vectors for rejuvenation with mono threads.

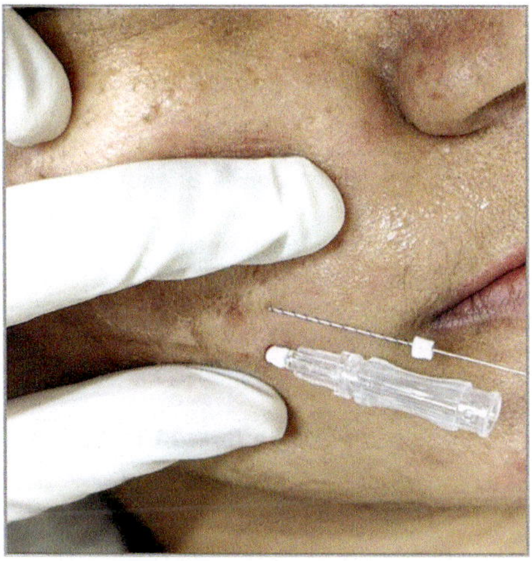

FIG. 7: Method of insertion of mono threads.

- The track of the needle should be visible, but the needle should not be visible.
- When the whole needle has gone in, screw it once and take out the needle.
- Check the opening for any protruding thread, which usually does not happen if the thread has been inserted correctly.
- In case, there is a protruding visible thread, either push it in or cut it.

HISTOLOGICAL CHANGES AFTER MONO THREAD INSERTION

- Tissue contraction by myofibroblast
- Newly formed fibrotic tissue
- Fat cell denaturation
- Increase in capillary size

CLINICAL PEARL

- Mono threads in combination with other procedures such as cog threads, skin boosters, fillers, and platelet-rich plasma give promising results.

CONCLUSION

Mono threads are a versatile and minimally invasive option in esthetic Dermatology offering subtle yet effective skin rejuvenation and tightening. While mono threads may not provide the lifting effect of cog or barbed threads, their safety profile and adaptability for various facial and body areas make them a valuable tool in our hands.

REFERENCES

1. Khattab FM, Samir MA, El Khouly SS, Atwa EM. Efficacy of Polycaprolactone Threads in Treating Atrophic Acne Scars: A Split-face Comparative Study. J Clin Aesthet Dermatol. 2023;16(9):33-7.
2. Arora G, Arora S. Periorbital Rejuvenation: A Study on the Use of Dermal Threads as Monotherapy, with a Review of Literature. J Cutan Aesthet Surg. 2022;15(1):48-57.
3. Metwalli M, Khattab FM, Mandour S. Monofilament threads in treatment of female hair loss. J Dermatolog Treat. 2021;32(5):521-5.
4. Dominguez-Santas M, Diaz-Guimaraens B, Saceda-Corralo D, Hermosa-Gelbard A, Muñoz-Moreno Arrones O, Pindado-Ortega C, et al. The state-of-the-art in the management of androgenetic alopecia: a review of new therapies and treatment algorithms. JEADV Clin Pract. 2022;1:176-85.
5. Arora G, Arora S. Neck Rejuvenation with Thread Lift. J Cutan Aesthet Surg. 2019;12(3): 196-200.
6. Procedure for treatment of abdominal skin. In: Kim NM (Ed). Non-Surgical Thread Procedures. Cham: Springer; 2023.

CHAPTER 6

Barbed Threads: Uses and Insertion

Indu Ballani, Aishwarya Raheja

INTRODUCTION

Barbed threads or cog threads are nonsmooth threads with small projections called barbs radiating from the center of thread. The barbs anchor to the tissues providing a firm grip (anchorage effect). These threads are known for their strong mechanical/lifting effect.[1]

USES OF COG THREADS

- *Facial rejuvenation*: Barbed threads improve the facial appearance by immediately lifting and tightening the sagged facial tissues.[1-4]
- *Jawline definition*: Cog threads when inserted along the jawline, give a good jawline definition and also improves the jowl and marionette lines.
- *Nose lift*: Lifting the nose with cog threads is an effective nonsurgical method of correcting nasal morphology defects such as concave nasal dorsum, dropped nasal tip, hanging columella, and nasolabial angle correction.[5]
- *Eyebrow lift*: For this indication, smaller cog threads are used. They are very helpful in lifting the lateral portion of the brows, which droops with age.[6]
- *Other indications*: Cog threads can also be used for treatment of skin problems such as stretch marks, scars, cellulite, and alopecia.

CLASSIFICATION OF COG THREADS

- *Based on the material*: PDO (polydioxanone)/P(LA/CL) (poly-L-lactic acid and caprolactone), PLLA (poly-L-lactic acid) threads are not available in India.
- *Based on the length*: Mentioned in **Table 1**.

TABLE 1: Length of cog threads and indications.

Length of cannula	Indication
6–8 cm	Nose and eyebrow
8–10 cm	Eyebrow and Jawline
10–12 cm	Mid-face, jowls, and neck

PROCEDURE FOR INSERTION OF BARBED THREADS

1. *Mark the vectors*: Vectors are marked depending on the target area **(Fig. 1)**.
2. *Anesthesia*: Lidocaine with adrenaline is preferred to reduce the chances of bleeding. Around 0.25 mL is injected at the entry point; 0.1 mL can be given at the zygomatic arch; and 0.1 mL at the end of the vector.

   Exorbitant amount of anesthesia should not be injected as it may increase swelling later on.

> CLINICAL PEARL
>
> If our cannula is in right layer (subcutaneous), it is usually not very painful. When the cannula is too superficial or deep, the patient may wince, thus guiding us whenever the layer goes wrong.

3. *Creating the entry point*: Entry point is created vertically with an 18-gauge needle going as deep as the bevel of the needle to reach the subcutaneous layer by pinching it **(Fig. 2)**.
4. *Inserting the cannula*: Pinch the entry point that you have created and insert the cannula vertically holding it like a pen. After screwing it in, you will feel a

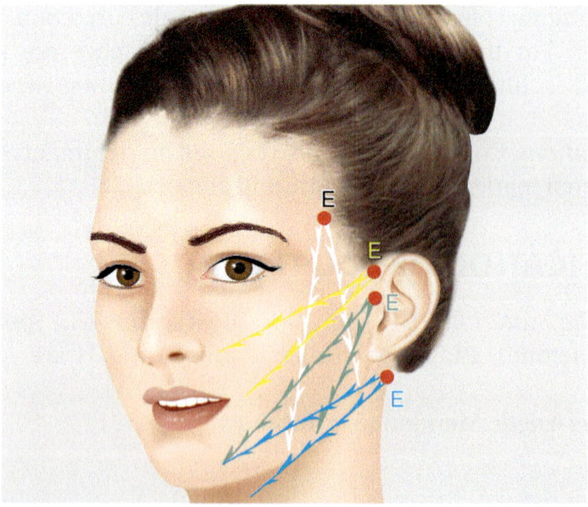

FIG. 1: Vectors for barbed threads.

bounce effect as the superficial musculoaponeurotic system (SMAS) is a thick layer. The cannula almost stands at this point. If it is superficial, the bevel comes out partially when you leave it.

5. *Pinching technique*: Once you have inserted the cannula into the subcutaneous at the entry point, start going horizontally along the planned vector pinching along the tract and making a passage for the cannula to slide into the subcutaneous **(Figs. 3A and B)**.

   It is important to shift your pinch ahead of the advancing canula so that a passage is created for a smooth insertion.

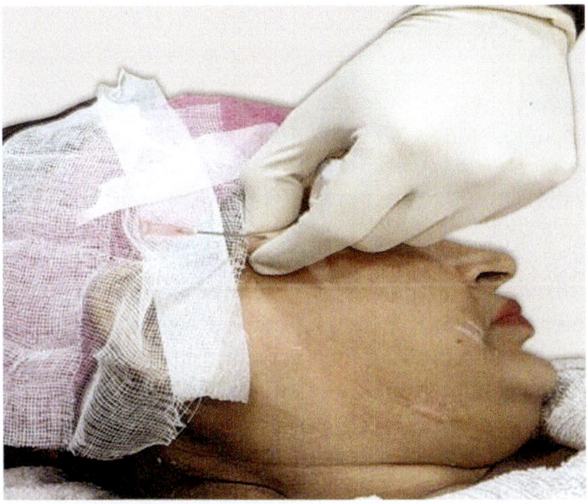

FIG. 2: Creating the entry point.

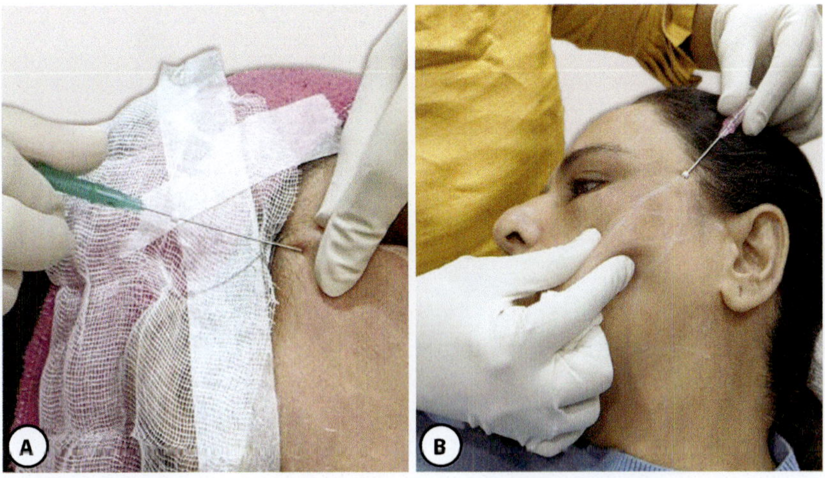

FIGS. 3A AND B: Pinching technique.

CLINICAL PEARL

We tend to become a bit superficial as the cannula advances. To prevent this, we can lift the hub of cannula as we move forward, so that the end goes into the deep subcutaneous.

6. *Inserting the second thread*: At the time of insertion of the second thread through the same entry point, move the projecting thread aside and insert the other cannula through the same point vertically just like the first thread and insert it in a similar manner **(Fig. 4)**.
7. *Pulling and intertwining the threads together*: Once the threads are inserted, we pull up the fat pads along the threads and open up the barbs by pressing along the tract in an upward direction. Both the threads are then pulled up and intertwined **(Fig. 5)**.

CLINICAL PEARLS

- Tying a knot is not preferred as that might cause projecting of the barb upwards as a nodule, if the knot is not embedded deep enough.
- Intertwining the barbs is a better option as it gives a good anchoring to the threads and works like a knot.

8. *Cutting the thread*: Both the threads are then pulled up and cut very close to the skin preferably with the tip of a curved scissors **(Fig. 6)**. After cutting a dimple is visible, slide the skin over this dimple, so that the barbs slip inside.

   The correct sequence is: Pull the thread, cut the thread by pressing the skin down, and then slide the skin over the entry point.
9. *Last step*: After cutting the thread, once again take your hand along the thread tract to open up and settle down the barbs. You will hear a sound of sliding barbs when they are settling inside. Apply a topical antibiotic at the entry point.

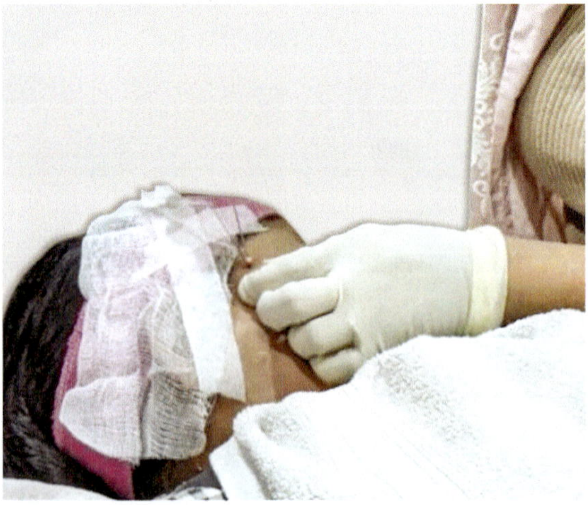

FIG. 4: Inserting the second thread.

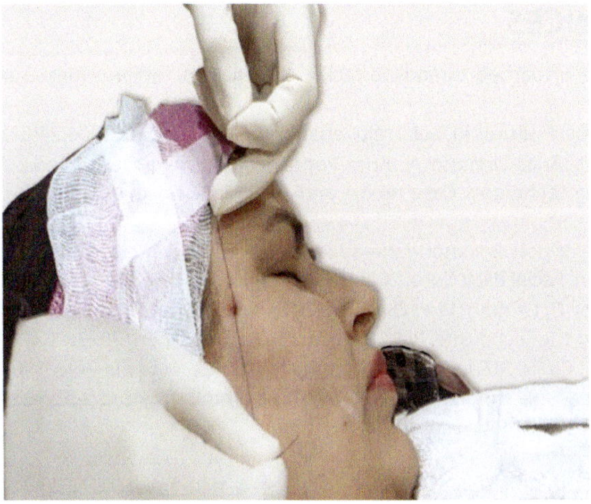

FIG. 5: Pulling and intertwining the threads.

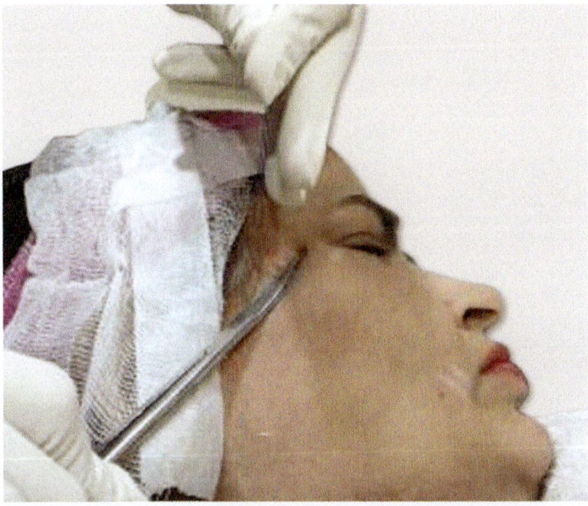

FIG. 6: Cutting the thread.

CLINICAL PEARL

It is always better that after completing one side, you ask the patient to sit and compare the two sides.

CONCLUSION

The unique design of barbed threads featuring hooks or barbs along the whole length of thread, provides immediate mechanical lifting while simultaneously stimulating collagen production for long-term rejuvenation.

Barbed threads are particularly effective in addressing sagging skin in midface, jawline and neck making them a popular procedure for natural looking results with minimum downtime.

REFERENCES

1. Kalra R. Use of barbed threads in facial rejuvenation. Indian J Plast Surg. 2008;41(Suppl): S93-S100.
2. Wu WT. Barbed sutures in facial rejuvenation. Aesthet Surg J. 2004;24(6):582-7.
3. Contreras C, Ariza-Donado A, Ariza-Fontalvo A. Using PDO threads: A scarcely studied rejuvenation technique. Case report and systematic review. J Cosmet Dermatol. 2023;22: 2158-65.
4. Cobo R. Use of polydioxanone threads as an alternative in non-surgical procedures in facial rejuvenation. Facial Plast Surg. 2020;36(4):447-52.
5. Sulamanidze C, Lanfranchi L, Diaspro A. Thread Lifting of the Nose: Fully Comprehensive Approach to the Technique. Plast Reconstr Surg Glob Open. 2023;11(4):e4907.
6. Santorelli A, Cirillo P, Fundarò SP, Cavallini M, Salti G, Avvedimento S. Eyebrow lifting with barbed threads: A simple, safe, and effective ambulatory procedure. J Cosmet Dermatol. 2023;22(1):140-5.

CHAPTER 7

Treating the Upper Face with Threads

Indu Ballani

INTRODUCTION

Forehead skin is the thinnest when compared to the rest of the face and tends to become thinner with age. The most common concerns in the upper face or the forehead area are skin laxity, loss of volume, and gradual descent of soft tissues, which leads to ptosis of the eyebrows. Brow ptosis occurs more on lateral side, hence this is the part which is targeted with threads to lift the eyebrows.[1,2] Mono threads can be used to improve the appearance of fine lines and improve the skin elasticity. Before planning any procedure, following classification should be kept in mind **(Fig. 1)**.

TYPES OF THREADS

- PDO (polydioxanone) cog threads 19 gauge.
- *PCL (polycaprolactone) cog or double needle*: Definisse/Silhouette soft/APTOS (Anti-Ptosis Suture)

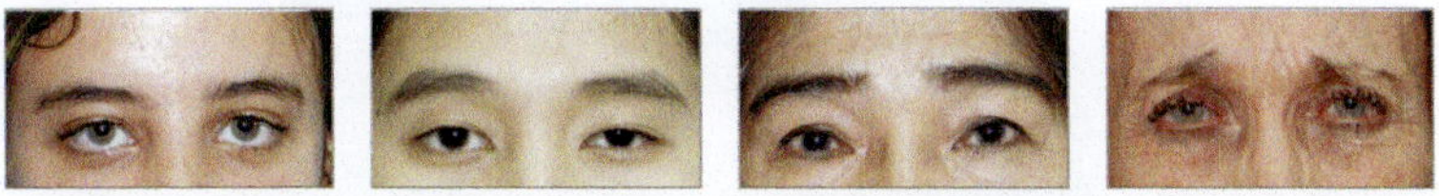

Unattractive	Tired	Aging	Sad
The middle third of the brow is at the same level than the medial third	Middle third of the brow is lower than the medial third	Lateral third of the brow is at the same level than the middle third	Lateral third of the brow is lower than the middle third
Therapeutic approach			
Lift	Relax + lift	Restore + lift	Restore + relax + lift
Main treatment			
Thread	BTXA + thread	Filler + threads	Filler + BTXA + thread

FIG. 1: Eyebrow classification.
Courtesy: Relife.

COUNSELING

Patient should be assessed whether the droop is in the eyebrows or the eyelids. Consideration should be given to the double eyelid lines, which develop in older age group due to laxity of the eyelid skin, this may not improve with lifting of eyebrows in this age group.

Normal or thick skin in the temporal area is also required as thin skin or hollowness in temples can pose a problem at the time of the insertion.

> CLINICAL PEARL
>
> The results of eyebrow lift are usually not very long lasting. Using newer methods of insertion like reverse vectors and combination treatments can increase the longevity.

ANATOMICAL CONSIDERATIONS

The supratrochlear and supraorbital artery arise from their respective foramen at the superior orbital rim and then become superficial in the upper two-thirds of the forehead.

Keeping this in mind, our threads should be in the subcutaneous layer in the lower third of forehead, but should be deeper in the supraperiosteal plane in upper two-thirds. Also, avoid inserting any thread in the medial part due to the risk of injuring these vessels or nerves.

VECTORS FOR INSERTION

- *Cog threads*: Reverse vectors are preferable. When the arch needs more prominence, two vectors from the high point of arch are preferred as shown in **Figure 2**. If the whole lateral part of eyebrow needs a lift, then two separate vectors can be chosen as shown in **Figure 3**.

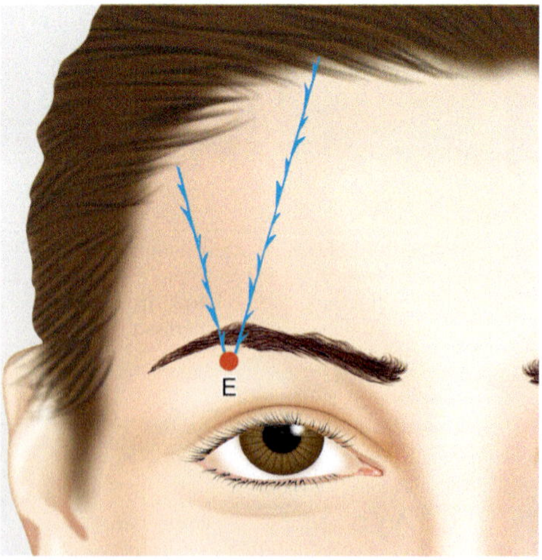

FIG. 2: Preferred vector to give high arch.

A better result would be achieved if all four vectors are done. The medial limit of the vectors is the supratrochlear notch beyond which the risk of injury to vasculature increases. The lateral limit is the temporal crest as there is thick tissue over here with the neurovascular bundles.

Fox tail eyebrow—this trend has gained a lot of popularity in the recent years. Fox tail eyebrow is an upward and outward sweeping shape of the eyebrow resembling the tail of a fox. The vectors used are described in **Figure 4**. These vectors also help in lifting the lateral part of the eyebrow. However, it is essential to consider individual anatomy and facial shape to ensure a natural and aesthetic result.

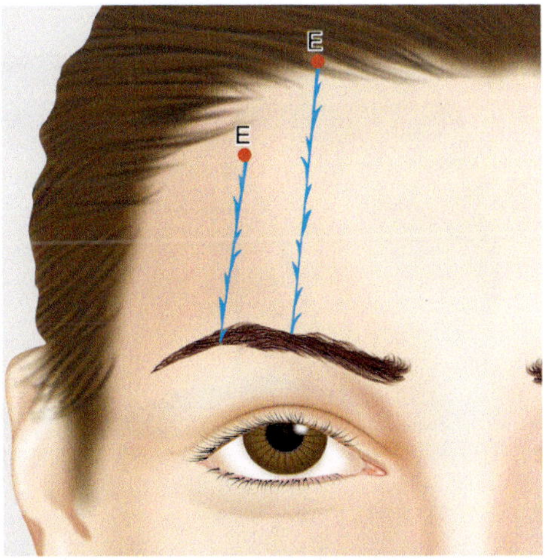

FIG. 3: Preferred vector for lateral lift of eyebrow.

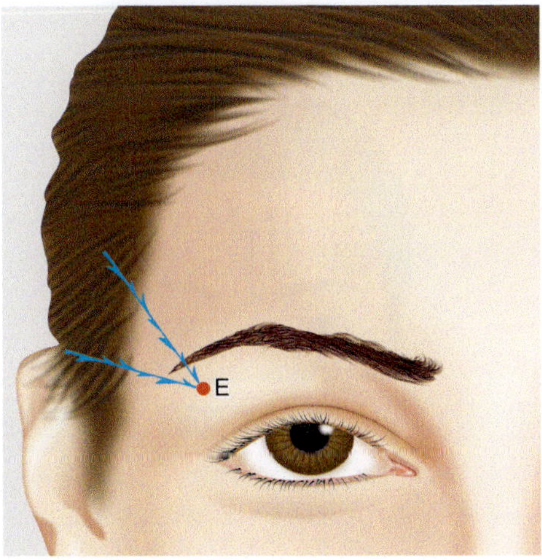

FIG. 4: Foxtail eyebrow.

- *Bidirectional needle threads*: If bidirectional needle threads are used, the point of insertion should be taken at the hairline as shown in **Figure 5**.[1] Also, U-shaped vector can be chosen instead of V.
- *Mono threads*: Small mono threads (25 mm or 38 mm) can be inserted in a meshwork pattern to improve the fine lines in the forehead area as shown in **Figure 6**.

THREAD INSERTION

- Giving lidocaine with adrenaline all along the tract helps in hydrodissection, which helps in easier passage of the thread.

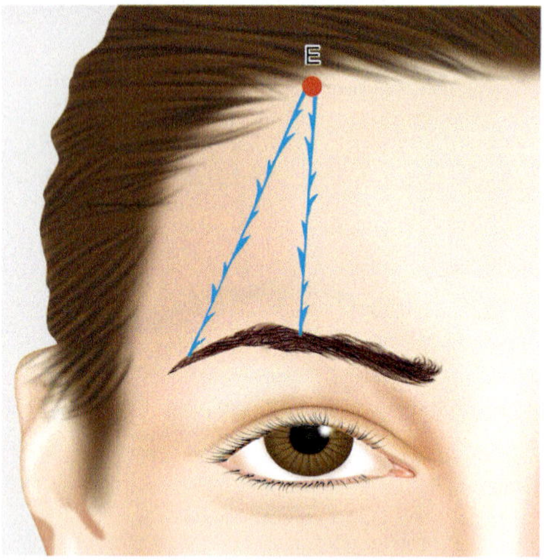

FIG. 5: Bidirectional needle threads.

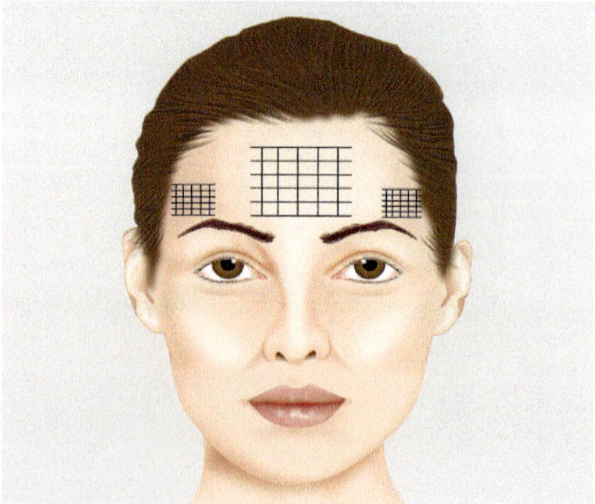

FIG. 6: Vectors for mono threads.

- It is difficult to follow the pinching technique in the forehead, but pinching should be done near the eyebrow and lower third of the forehead, so that the subcutaneous depth is maintained **(Figs. 7 and 8)**.
- Thread should be cut very close to the skin being careful of the eyebrow hair, after pulling the threads upward and toward the hairline **(Fig. 9)**.

COMPLICATIONS

- *Bleeding*: It can occur due to the rich vasculature, especially at entry point. Use of lidocaine with adrenaline can minimize the risk of bleeding. Bruising if occurs may take 2 weeks to resolve **(Figs. 10A and B)**.

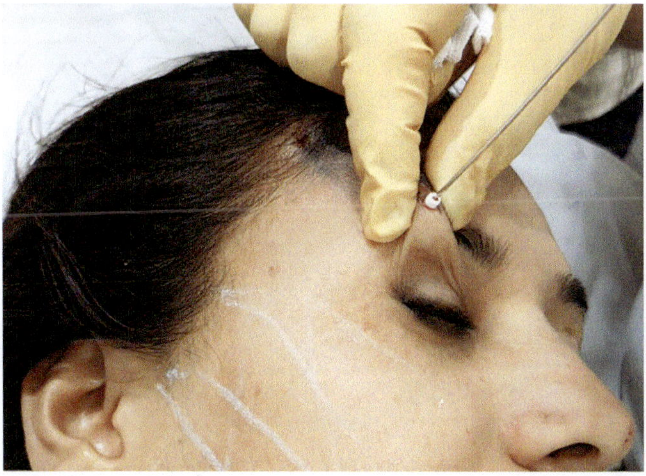

FIG. 7: Entry point.

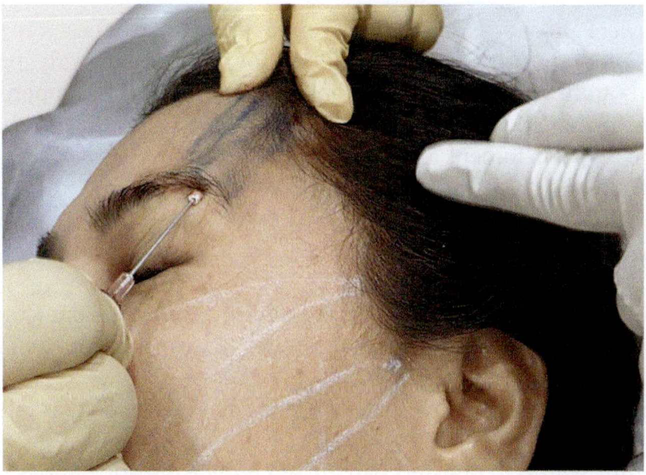

FIG. 8: Pinching technique.

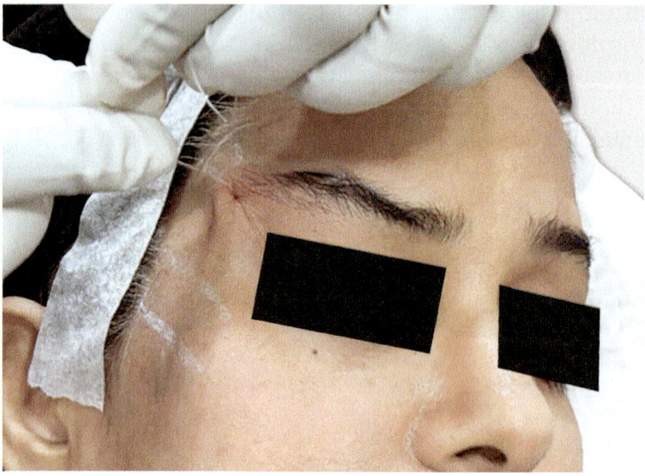

FIG. 9: Pulling the threads.

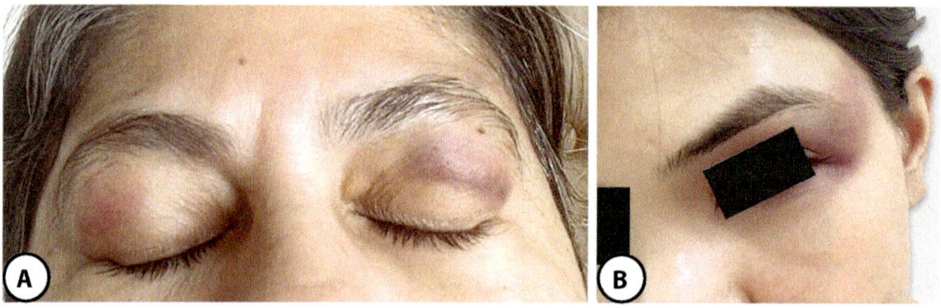

FIGS. 10A AND B: Bruising at the procedure site.

- *Headache*: Pain or swelling can happen for around 2 weeks.
- *Protrusion of the barb*: If the thread has not been cut properly, projection of the barb at the entry point might pose a problem. If this happens, the entry point is freshened with an 18-gauge needle, the protruding barb is grasped with the help of a forceps and cut **(Fig. 11)**.
  Figs. 10A and B: Bruising at the procedure site.

OTHER CONSIDERATIONS

- Combining it with procedures like Botulinum toxin for relaxing the muscle is recommended. In fact, the result of eyebrow lift can stay longer if the toxin is repeated every 4 months **(Fig. 12)**.[1]
- Adding volume to a hollow or concave forehead is also advisable for better results.
- Combining with skin boosters can further reduce the appearance of fine lines and improve the skin elasticity.

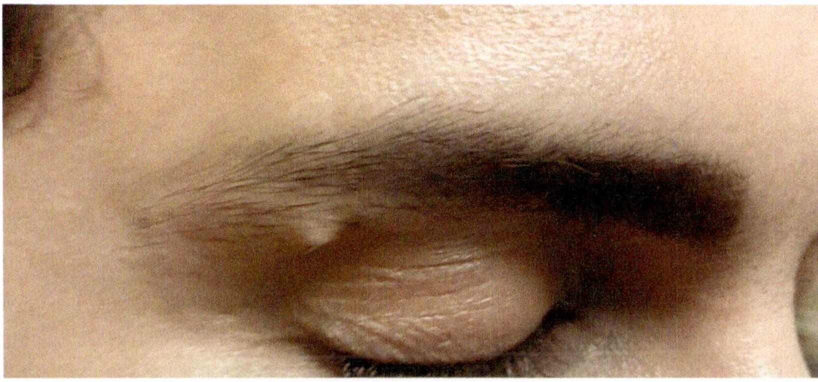

FIG. 11: Protrusion of the barb.

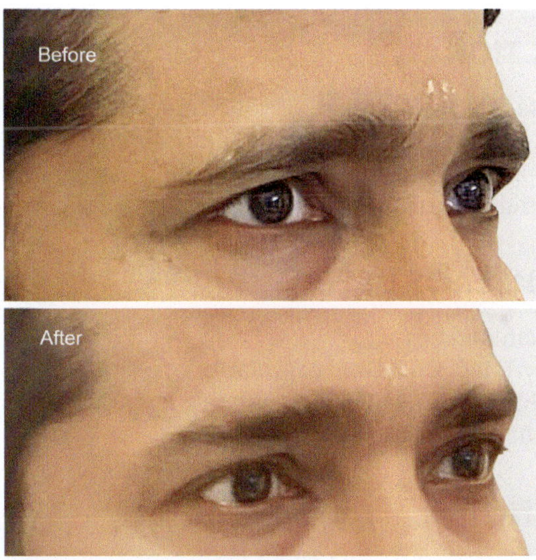

FIG. 12: Results of eyebrow cog threads.

CONCLUSION

Eyebrow thread lifting has emerged as a highly effective technique for achieving a more defines and youthful brow. It is a very useful procedure for prevention of drooping due to the mechanical lifting and collagen stimulation provided by threads and can also address brow asymmetry to a certain extent.

REFERENCES

1. Santorelli A, Cirillo P, Fundarò SP, Cavallini M, Salti G, Avvedimento S. Eyebrow lifting with barbed threads: A simple, safe, and effective ambulatory procedure. J Cosmet Dermatol. 202;22(1):140-5.
2. Kim H, Jung J, Choi SW, Yun CW, Lee W. Eyebrow lifting using multidirectional absorbable thread. J Cosmet Dermatol. 2023;22(10):2780-4.

CHAPTER 8

Treating the Mid Face with Threads

Indu Ballani

INTRODUCTION

A volumized midface is the hallmark of youthfulness, and it is the first area to show visible signs of aging. Threads play an important role in lifting the malar fat pads and improving the nasolabial folds. When there is volume loss in the deep fat pads, combination treatment with fillers gives better outcome.

TYPE OF THREADS USED

- PDO (polydioxanone) cog
- P(LA/CL) (poly-L-lactic acid and caprolactone) cog
- P(LA/CL) double needle (MR technique)
- P(LA/CL) free floating threads

COUNSELING

- Lifting the mid-face and nasolabial folds is important to show an improvement in under eye area or before filling the nasolabial **(see Fig. 5)**.
- Some patients who do not prefer chubby cheeks or filled cheek appearance with fillers may go in for lifting of the nasolabial folds.
- If anteromedial cheek projection is required, the Definisse free floating threads may be used as they are ideal for malar reshaping and projection **(see Fig. 6)**.

ANATOMY

The zygomatic ligament is strongly attached to the deep fascia. Hence, sometimes there is some resistance felt when passing the thread through this area. The entry point should be such that the thread hooks through it for a good tightening result.

CLINICAL PEARL

The nasolabial folds should not be crossed with threads as the nasolabial skin is thin and the facial artery is in subcutaneous layer in the upper part of nasolabial fold.

VECTORS FOR INSERTION CANNULA THREADS

The threads for nasolabial folds are inserted in a V shape with entry point near tragus of ear or higher and the two vectors going on to nose and angle of mouth but stopping just before the fold.

V-SHAPED VECTORS

- *Cannula threads*: Usually when two cannula threads are inserted from or above the zygomatic arch toward the nasolabial fold through a single entry point, a good lift can be obtained.
- *Double needle P(LA/CL) threads*: Double needle PLCL [poly(L-lactide-Co-ε-caprolactone)] thread can also be inserted in a similar manner like cannula threads with both needles inserted along the 2 vectors **(Fig. 1)**.
- Aptos threads are a type of P(LA/CL) multidirectional cutting threads in which a 20-gauge cannula is used to insert multiple threads from one entry point to increase the lifting effect as shown in **Figure 2**.

Reverse vectors are special vectors for uplifting the cheek and eyebrow region.

As the name implies, these vectors start from the cheek and are inserted in a reverse direction toward the scalp. This utilizes the whole length of the thread and anchors it in the temporal fascia, which has dense reticulation, hence leads to better anchoring **(Fig. 3)**.

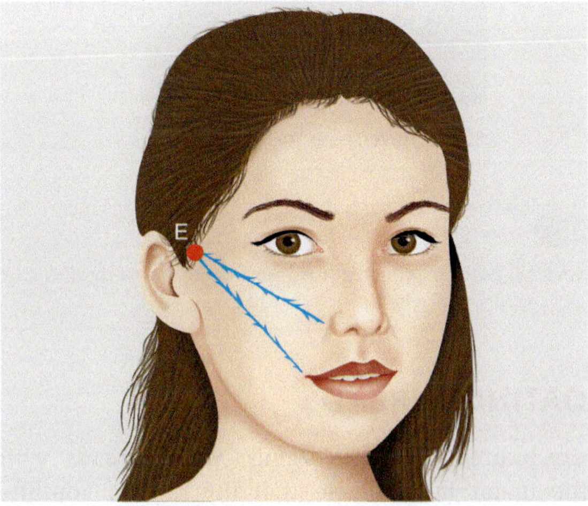

FIG. 1: Cog threads.

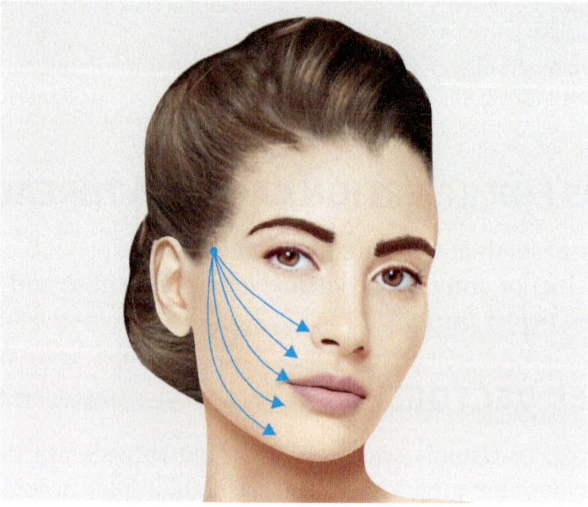

FIG. 2: Vectors of Aptos threads.

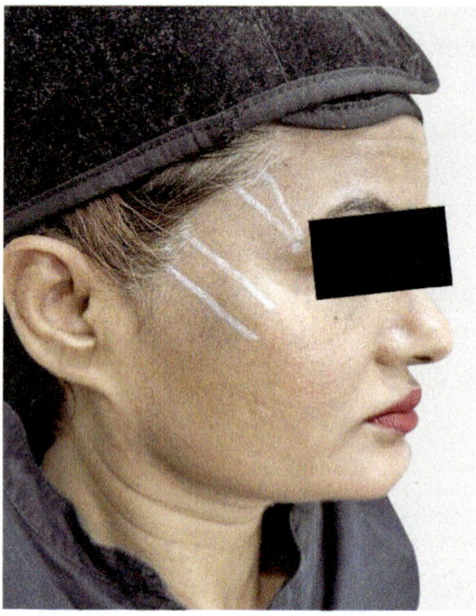

FIG. 3: Reverse vectors.

CLINICAL PEARL

Face may look wider if assessment has not been done properly and the vertical temple vector is not done simultaneously.

FREE FLOATING THREADS

These threads are bidirectional converging type of threads, which are used for repositioning the malar fat pads, so that the natural youthful anteromedial cheek projection is regained **(see Fig. 6)**.[1] The technique is known as "soft tissue reshaping" or STR 2 (when 2 threads are used per side) and STR 3 (when 3 threads

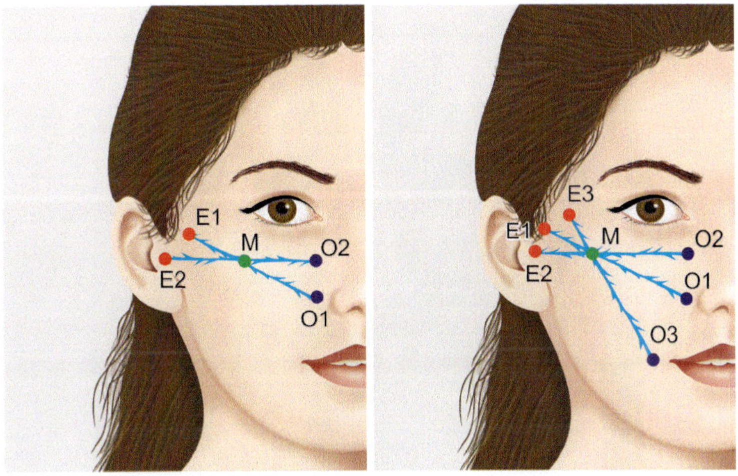

FIG. 4: Free floating threads for volumizing mid cheek.

are used per side). The threads are inserted through a 20-gauge spinal cannula with entry and exit points as shown in **Figure 4**. Available length of the thread in India is 12 cm.

THREAD INSERTION

The malar fat pads are usually bulky in Indians and a curvature has to be followed while inserting the threads. Hence, a wide pinch along the tract and lifting the end of the cannula at the entry point helps in advancing the thread in a proper layer.

COMPLICATIONS

- A barb may be visible as a nodule at the thread end inside nasolabial fold (NLF). This happens when we cross the NLF with the threads.
- Bruising is common when needle threads are used.

OTHER CONSIDERATIONS

If during assessment we feel that a combination treatment with fillers may be required for giving cheek projection, then free floating threads provide a good alternative for a natural look with slight cheek projection and lifting. A nasolabial filler may still be required if volume loss is visible even after lifting.

RESULTS

Results of eight cog threads and three pairs of free floating threads are shown in **Figures 5 and 6**.

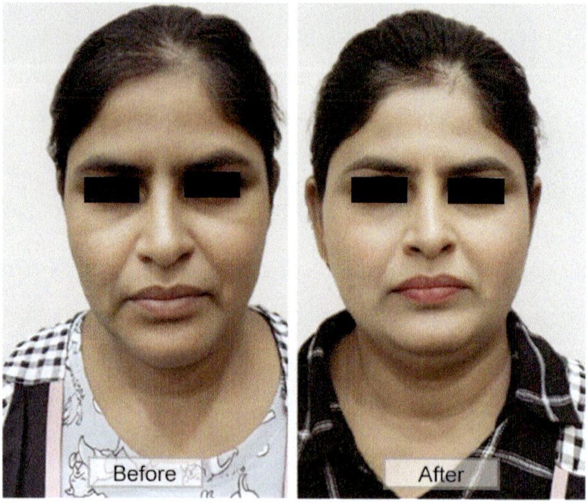

FIG. 5: Result of eight cog threads for mid face.

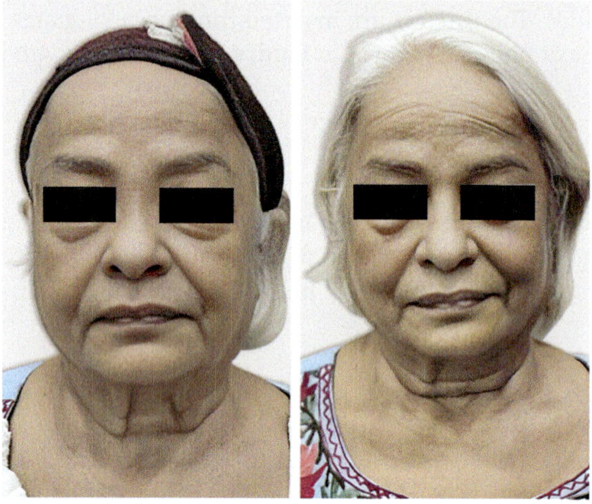

FIG. 6: Result of three pairs of free floating threads in a 67-year-old woman.

CONCLUSION

Threads provide a natural lifting effect by repositioning tissues and stimulating collagen production without adding excessive bulk. This makes them an ideal choice for redefining midface contours, softening nasolabial folds and restoring youthful proportions when compared to fillers.

REFERENCE

1. Santorelli A, Cerullo F, Cirillo P, Cavallini M, Avvedimento S. Mid-face reshaping using threads with bidirectional convergent barbs: A retrospective study. J Cosmet Dermatol. 2021;20(6):1591-7.

CHAPTER 9

Nose Reshaping with Threads

Indu Ballani

INTRODUCTION

The nose is a central and defining feature of the face. A sharp upturned nose is a desirable feature, and threads are an easy nonsurgical option for sharpening it. They can be used to correct the nasal morphology defects like concave nasal dorsum, dropped nasal tip, and wide nostrils.[1] **Figure 1** can be used as an assessment guide for the nose threads.

NOSE TIP PTOSIS CLASSIFICATION

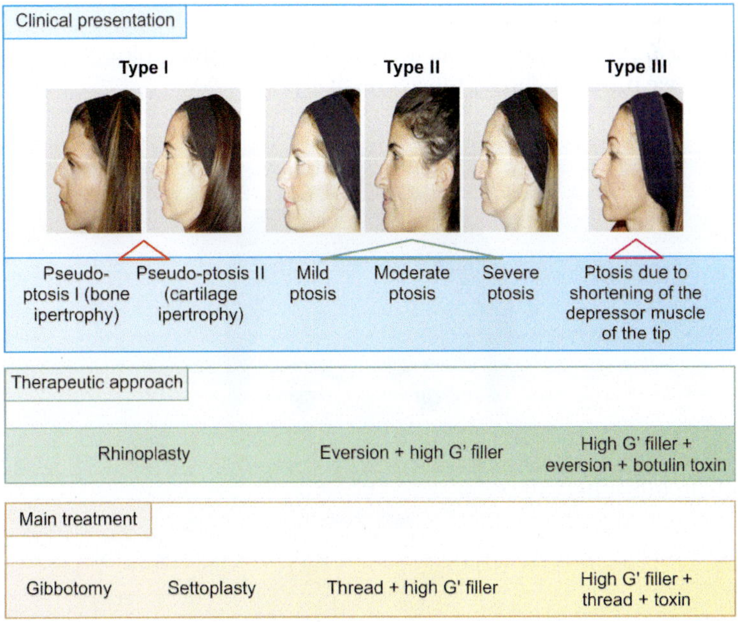

FIG. 1: Classification and images of Dr A Santorelli.
Courtesy: Relife.

TYPES OF THREADS USED

- PDO (polydioxanone) cog threads
- PCL (polycaprolactone) cog threads

ANATOMICAL CONSIDERATIONS

Avoid injury to the alar artery, a branch of the nasal artery at the root of nose and the columellar artery at the columella as these give small branches, which directly supply the eyeball.

CLINICAL PEARL

The nose is a highly vascular structure with superficial vessels anastomosing all around. Therefore, level of insertion for threads is perichondrial or periosteum.

VECTORS FOR INSERTION

Entry point is taken at tip of nose between the two alar cartilages or domes, and four cannula threads are inserted above or alongside each other after injecting the local anesthesia **(Figs. 2 and 3)**.

Four cannula threads along columella down to nasal spine help in further elevating the tip **(Table 1 and Fig. 4)**. Result can be seen in **Figures 5A and B**.

COMPLICATIONS

- Pain and swelling might last up to a week.
- *Vascular injury*: Since nose is a highly vascular area, injury to vessels can occur if we push the thread too aggressively.

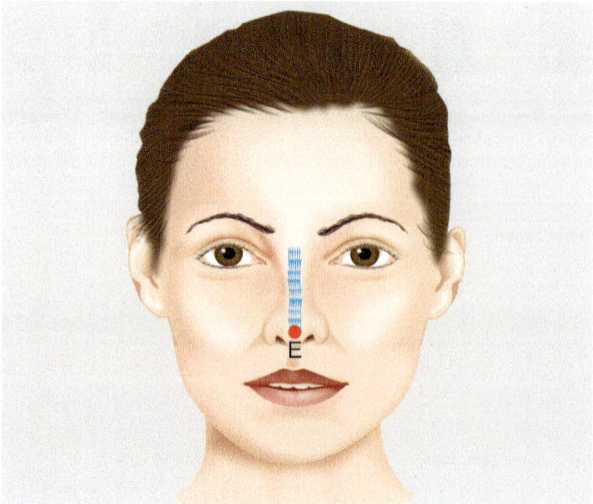

FIG. 2: Vectors for nasal bridge.

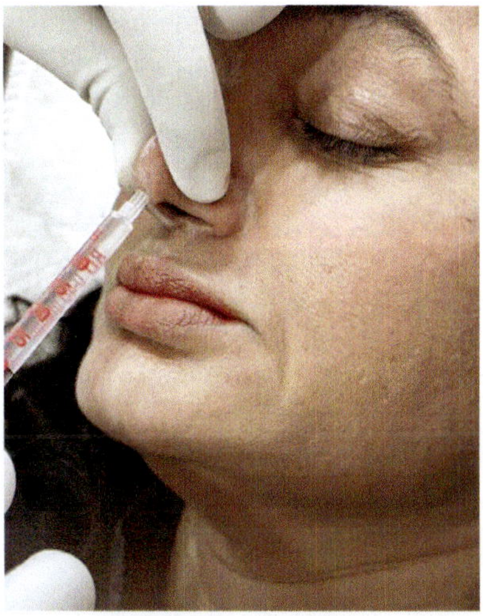

FIG. 3: Injecting the local anesthesia.

TABLE 1: Length of nose threads and indications.

Site	Length of the thread	Indication
Nasal dorsum	9.5 cm	To sharpen the nasal bridge
Columella	6 cm	To elevate the nasal tip

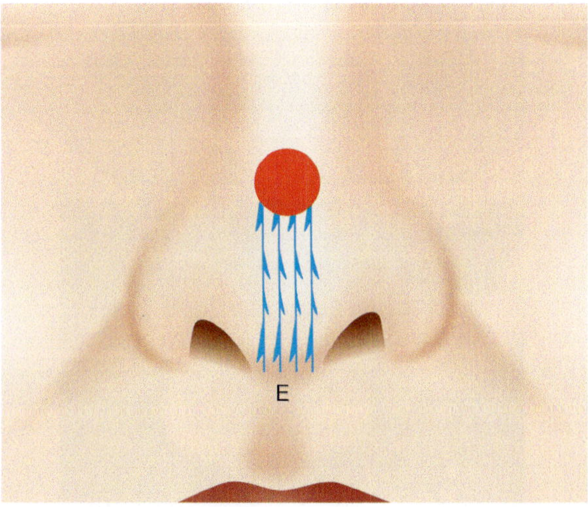

FIG. 4: Vector for columella.

- *Extrusion of the thread*: PDO cog threads used for nose are very thick and sometimes, a tiny part of the thread may extrude from the entry point. This can be avoided by pushing the thread inside while cutting.
- Superficial placement of the thread **(Fig. 6)**

CLINICAL PEARLS

- Local anesthesia should preferably be given at three points (nasal tip, midpoint of nasal bridge, and nasal root). This helps in hydrodissection, allowing easy passage of the thread **(Fig. 3)**.
- Combining with botulinum toxin, helps in further elevation of the nasal tip.

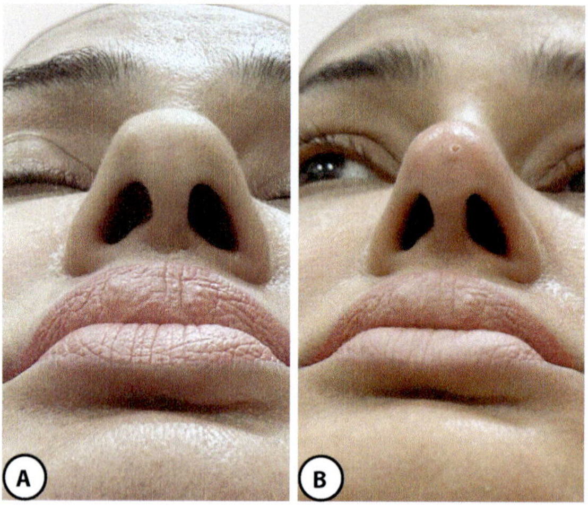

FIGS. 5A AND B: Result of nose thread.

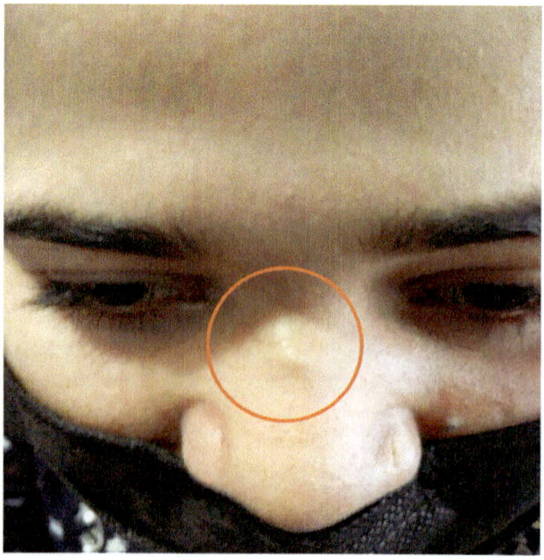

FIG. 6: Superficial placement of the thread.

CONCLUSION

Nose reshaping with threads offers a ground breaking, minimally invasive alternative to surgical rhinoplasty, making it an attractive option for patients seeking subtle yet effective enhancements. It is a safer otion with faster recovery and reduced complications as compared to fillers.

REFERENCE

1. Sulamanidze C, Lanfranchi L, Diaspro A. Thread Lifting of the Nose: Fully Comprehensive Approach to the Technique. Plast Reconstr Surg Glob Open. 2023;11(4):e4907.

CHAPTER 10

Treating the Lower Face with Threads

Indu Ballani

INTRODUCTION

Defined jawline is the hallmark of an attractive face. The demand for a better jawline is increasing in younger individuals also. Usually, threads give better results in the lower face compared to fillers because of their lifting effects.

TYPES OF THREADS

- PDO (polydioxanone) cog threads
- P(LA/CL) (poly-L-lactic acid and caprolactone) cog threads
- P(LA/CL) double needle threads

PATIENT SELECTION AND COUNSELING

Any person with signs of aging, descent of fat pads, deep marionettes, and visible jowls or softer jawline is a good candidate for jawline and lower face threads. Consideration should be given to a pre-existing genetically weak jawline where fillers are a better treatment.

ANATOMICAL CONSIDERATIONS

- For uplifting the jowls, a better anchoring point would be at the temple, thus giving it a good fixation in the temple area.
- The zygomatic ligament and the platysma-auricular ligament are other vectors that help in uplifting the jowls.
- When there is medial displacement of tissues, horizontal vectors along with temple vector are useful. For marionettes, oblique and vertical vectors are preferred.
- Pushing the thread too deep can cause complications related to the parotid gland and the fascia.

VECTORS FOR COG THREADS

- *Marionette vectors*: Entry point is taken at or above the tragus **(Fig. 1)**. This vector is preferred where marionette lines are deep.
- *Jawline vectors*: This vector is preferred where jawline is not defined and medial shift of tissues is visible. Good anchoring can be achieved by choosing entry point at platysma-auricular ligament. Single entry point or two entry points can be chosen **(Fig. 2)**.
- *Temple vectors*: These are the most preferred vectors for Indian faces and should be attempted before the jawline or marionette vectors, so that the upper part of face gets lifted first **(Fig. 3)**.

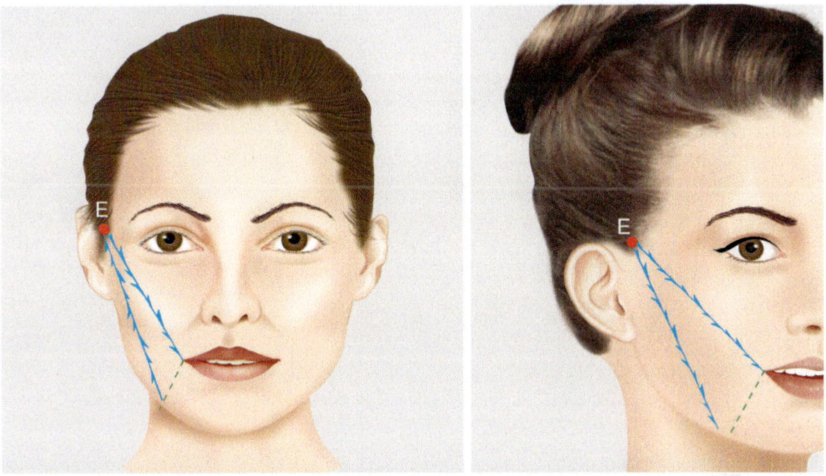

FIG. 1: Marionette vectors.

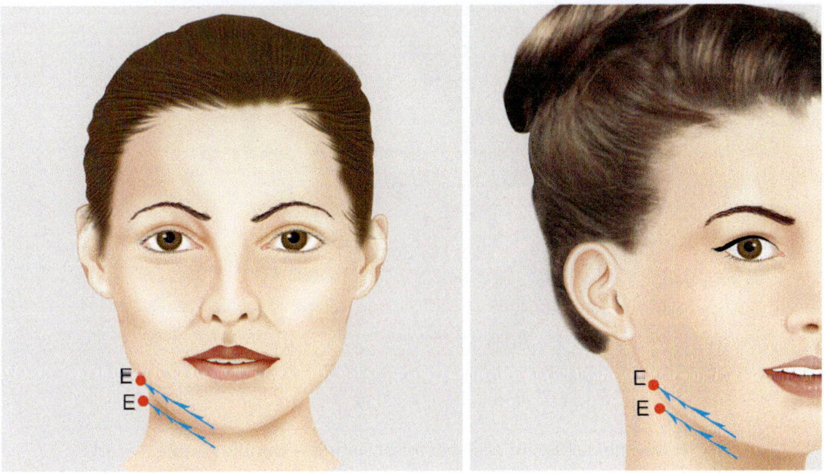

FIG. 2: Jawline vectors.

CLINICAL PEARL

Marionette line should not be crossed as the distal barbs of the thread might become visible as a bump during facial movements because of the thin skin in this area.

DOUBLE NEEDLE THREADS

Figure 4 shows the entry and exit points for double needle threads. The vector is called the jawline reshaping or JR vector for Definisse double needle threads.[1]

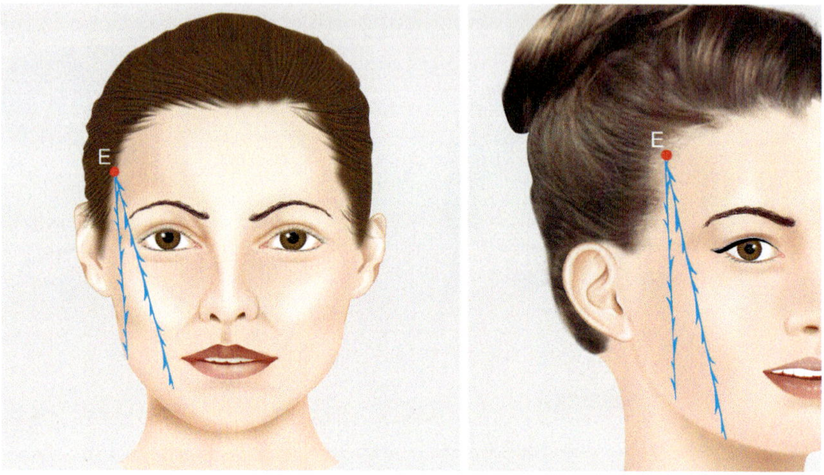

FIG. 3: Temple vectors.

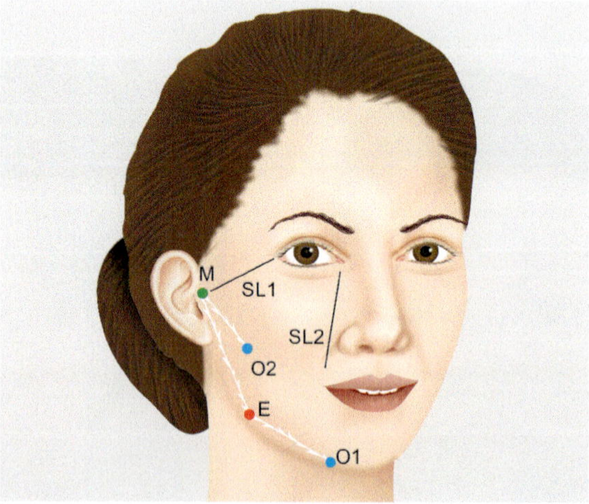

FIG. 4: Jawline reshaping or JR vector of Definisse double needle threads.

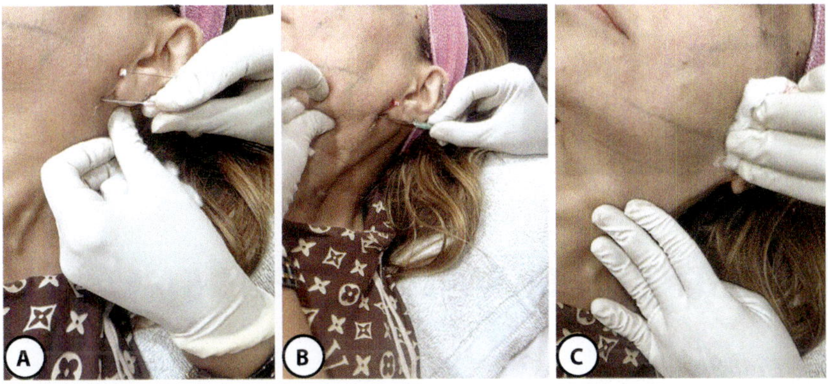

FIGS. 5A TO C: Insertion of thread along jawline.

THREAD INSERTION

Pinching technique throughout the tract of cannula aids in advancing the thread in correct layer **(Figs. 5A to C)**.

COMPLICATIONS

- Deeper penetration in the parotid area may cause complications related to the parotid gland like pain and swelling.
- If entry point is chosen near the mastoid process, it becomes difficult to maneuver the cannula along the jawline causing trauma to this area.

COMBINATION TREATMENTS

Better results are achieved with combination treatments. Combining threads with jawline and chin fillers may enhance the results. Nefertiti lift with botulinum toxin increases the longevity of the results.

CONCLUSION

As techniques and thread technology continue to evolve, lower face threads remain at the forefront of esthetic lifting treatments. They provide a reliable, safe and highly effective solution for achieving a youthful and well contoured appearance.

REFERENCE

1. Wanitphakdeedecha R, Yan C, Ng JNC, Fundarò S. Absorbable Barbed Threads for Lower Facial Soft-Tissue Repositioning in Asians. Dermatol Ther (Heidelb). 2021;11(4):1395-408.

CHAPTER 11

Treating Neck with Threads

Indu Ballani

INTRODUCTION

With the passage of time, neck is an area which shows a lot of sagging, especially because of the thin skin and soft tissues of this area. When the face has been treated with injectables and the neck is left untreated, the contrast becomes even more. Hence, it is very important to treat the neck along with the face to give a complete result.[1]

TYPES OF THREADS

- PDO (polydioxanone)/PCL (polycaprolactone) mono threads
- PDO/P(LA/CL) (poly-L-lactic acid and caprolactone) cog threads
- Double needle threads PDO/P(LA/CL)

PATIENT SELECTION AND COUNSELING

When patients are in their late 30s or 40s, they might just ask for a double chin treatment in heavier faces or else lines. Here comes the role of counseling and targeting the lower part of neck as well along with face treatments as it will be preventive. Mono threads, especially the P(LA/CL) threads, act as boosters to improve the quality of a wrinkly neck, but these should always be done after targeting the lateral part of neck with cog threads along the jawline.

ANATOMICAL CONSIDERATIONS

The thyroid gland and trachea are major structures located in the midline and as the skin of neck is thin, these may be at risk if our layer goes wrong. Hence, cog threads in the neck should be done with great caution and threads with finer gauge cannula should be preferred, especially when we are doing cog threads on lower part of neck. The thin skin of the neck makes it more prone to bruising even with mono threads. Direction of mono threads should be medial to lateral to be on a safer side.

VECTORS FOR INSERTION

- *Mono threads on neck* **(Figs. 1A and B)** can be inserted in any manner depending on the concerned area. Results are better if more number of threads are inserted.
- *Cog threads* can be inserted below the jawline. Two threads are inserted from a single opening **(Fig. 2)**. If entire neck has to be targeted, vectors described in **Figure 3** can be used.
- *Double needle threads*: The vectors for these can be the same as cog threads from a single opening (V vector) as described in **Figure 4** or U shape with an intermediate loop in between.

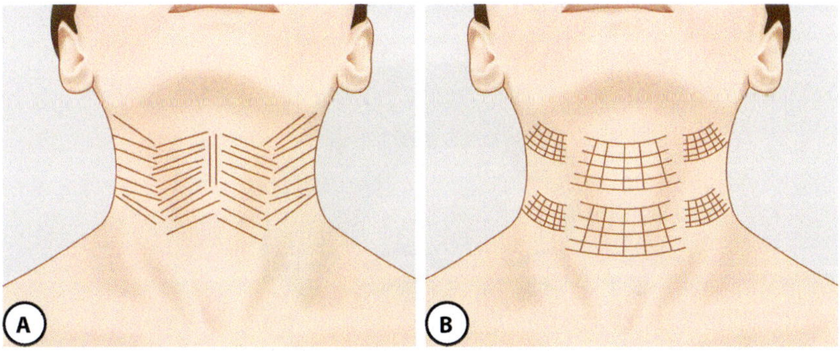

FIGS. 1A AND B: Vectors for mono threads.

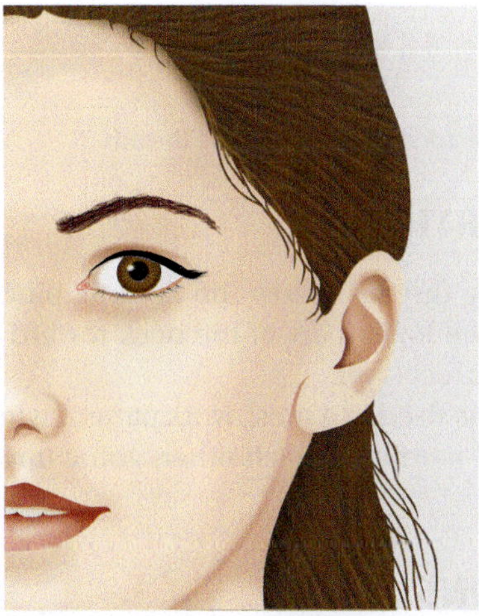

FIG. 2: Vectors for cog threads.

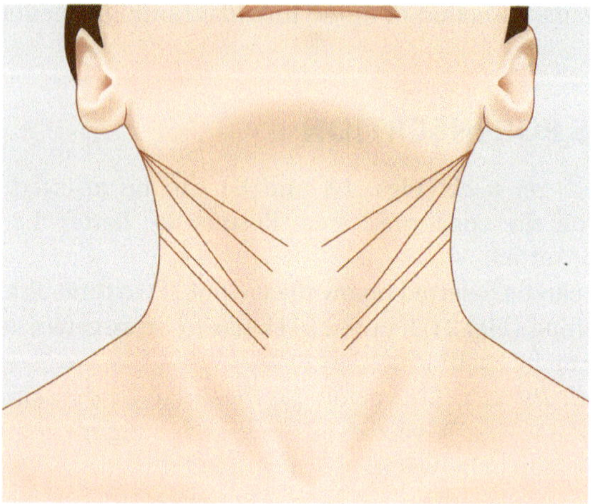

FIG. 3: Vectors for cog threads on entire neck.

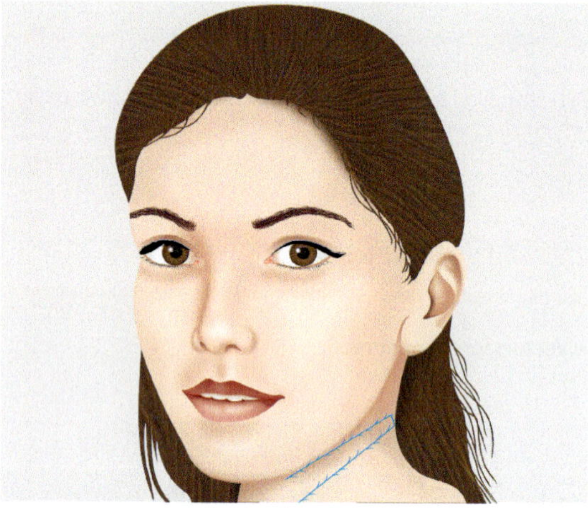

FIG. 4: Vectors for double needle threads.

THREAD INSERTION

While inserting the cog threads below the jawline, pinching becomes difficult, but we can pinch up the lower part of the neck toward the jawline, so that the thread can enter the correct layer.

Mono threads can be used in a meshwork pattern when improvement in skin quality is required and parallel to each other, going upward and laterally when lifting is required.

COMPLICATIONS

Bruising and hematoma formation are the most common complications in this area because of injury to superficial vessels.

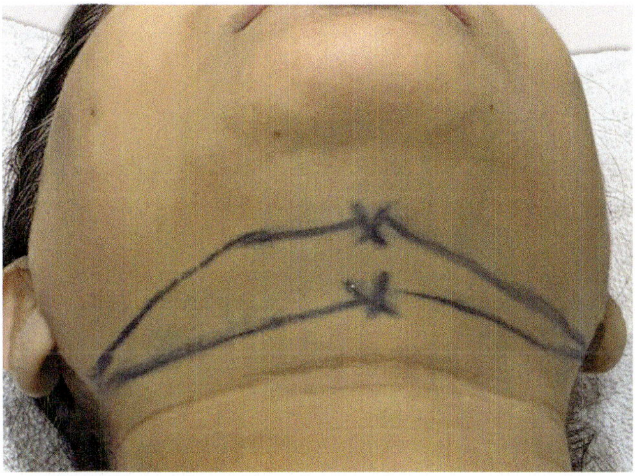

FIG. 5: Double needle threads for double chin.

OTHER CONSIDERATIONS

- Cog threads or double needle threads with entry from angle of mandible should be preferred when neck lifting is required.
- Double needle threads going from center to angle of mandible in a sling-like manner is preferred for heavy double chin as it repositions the fat more laterally **(Fig. 5)**.

Neck is an area which requires a lot of combination treatments for best results, and thread lift on neck is one of the important procedures for neck rejuvenation.

> CLINICAL PEARL
>
> Always begin by placing cog threads along the jawline and upper neck to address skin laxity before inserting mono threads. This approach follows the same principle as targeting the lateral areas of the face before treating the medial areas.

CONCLUSION

There are few effective nonsurgical options for neck laxity and sagging. Threads serve as an invaluable adjuvant treatment by proving an immediate lift. They complement other modalities such as energy based devices and injectables offering a comprehensive approach to neck rejuvenation.

REFERENCE

1. Hong GW, Kim SB, Park SY, Wan J, Yi KH. Basic concepts in facial and neck thread lifting procedures. Skin Res Technol. 2024;30(4):e13673.

CHAPTER 12

Postprocedure Care and Contraindications

Indu Ballani, Rashmi Sarkar

INTRODUCTION

After undergoing a thread-lift procedure, some specific postprocedure care needs to be followed by patients to optimize the results.

IMMEDIATE CARE

- Ice packs can be used to reduce swelling and pain.
- Avoid touching the area to prevent irritation or displacement.
- For double needle threads, Steri-Strips may be used for 48–72 hours postprocedure.

HOME CARE

- Patient is advised to avoid strenuous activities and high impact exercises for 5–7 days.
- Pain killers or anti-inflammatory tablets can be routinely prescribed for 3–5 days.
- Antibiotics may be prescribed if patient is diabetic or if the treating physician feels it is necessary.
- Vitamin supplements could be prescribed to promote good healing.
- Gentle skin care routine and avoiding vigorous scrubbing should be followed for 5–7 days.

The patient may be advised to sleep straight or with head elevated for 3–5 nights to minimize swelling and asymmetrical results due to pressure on one side.[1]

The patient should be advised to be regular with their sun protection using a good sun protection factor (SPF) to avoid any postinflammatory pigmentation on prick points.

Follow-up appointments should be given to monitor improvements.

CONTRAINDICATIONS

Although generally it is considered to be a safe procedure, there may be some contraindications, which make a patient unsuitable for the procedure.

- *Pregnancy and lactation*: These are usually absolute contraindications as the safety of any such procedures has not been established in these conditions.
- *Skin infections*: Active skin infections, such as acne and herpes, should be treated before performing the procedure.
- *Autoimmune conditions*: Patients with autoimmune conditions, such as arthritis or a compromised immune system, should be evaluated properly before considering them for a procedure.
- *Previous cosmetic procedures*: Patients who have had surgical or other injectable procedures (like permanent fillers) should be evaluated properly before proceeding with the treatments.
- *Unrealistic expectations*: Patients with unrealistic expectations or on psychiatric treatment are usually not good candidates for these procedures.

CLINICAL PEARL

- The safety and efficacy of our procedure can be enhanced by following proper guidelines and considering all the contraindications before planning the procedure.

CONCLUSION

Postprocedure care and contraindications is essential for ensuring safe and successful outcomes with thread lift treatments, proper aftercare plays a crucial role in optimizing results and minimizing complications. By prioritizing patient education and meticulous planning, thread lifts can be performed with confidence, delivering natural and effective results while maintaining highest standards of safety and patient satisfaction.

REFERENCE

1. Hong GW, Wan J, Yoon SE, Wong S, Yi KH. Pre- and Post-Procedural Considerations and Thread Types for Thread Lifting. Life. 2025;15(1):85.

CHAPTER 13

Other Types and Indications of Threads

Indu Ballani

INTRODUCTION

The field of thread based rejuvenation is still evolving and there is a wide array of thread types tailored to specific esthetic goals. Various other threads are expanding the scope of available treatments. This chapter delves into diverse type of threads and their indications, highlighting how they can be utilized for advanced facial and body rejuvenation.

TWIN SCREW THREADS

Twin screw threads are a type of smooth threads where two threads are wound around a needle usually 29 gauge 50 mm. Since more amount of material is being injected with these threads, the results are supposed to be slightly better than the simple mono threads used for rejuvenation.

TORNADO THREADS

Tornado threads are also a type of screw threads, which have small barbs but mounted on needles. They are used as an aid for jawline lifting along with cog threads or alone if only mild lifting is required.

CAVERN SCREW

Cavern screw are smaller smooth threads screwed around a needle inside a cannula for insertion **(Fig. 1)**. These threads give a good skin plumping up effect. They are inserted into the subcutaneous layer. The effects are maximized when multifill threads are used along with these.

Indications include forehead augmentation, glabella lines, eyebrow augmentation, under eye, cheekbones, nasolabial folds, and marionette lines.

MULTIFILL THREADS

Multifill threads are special monofilament threads for the nasolabial folds **(Fig. 2)**. As the name implies, these are multiple smooth threads on one needle injected along the nasolabial fold to give a smoothening effect. Other indications are forehead and eyebrow augmentation.

MOLDING MESH THREADS

Molding mesh threads are a variety of smooth threads, which are more powerful, strong, and long lasting. Main purpose is tightening and revitalization in areas like temple, cheeks, and heavy jaw.

SILHOUETTE SOFT THREADS

Silhouette soft is another PLLA (poly-l-lactic acid) thread, which has cones instead of barbs and is used for lifting and contouring the face.[1,2] It is manufactured by company Sinclair and was available in India earlier.

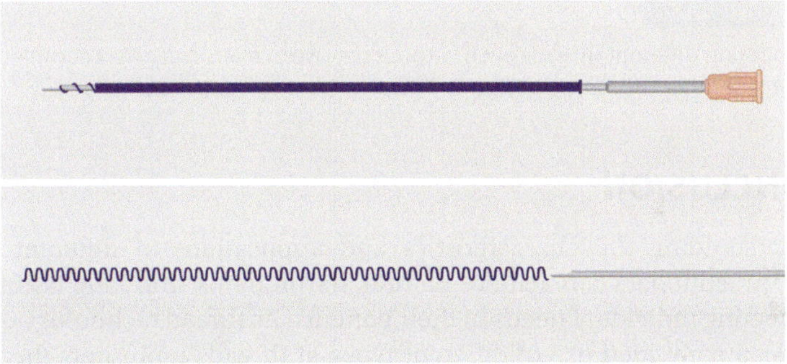

FIG. 1: Cavern screw threads.

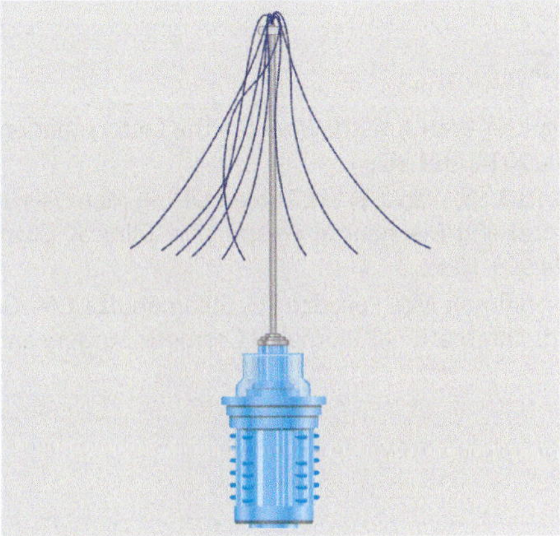

FIG. 2: Multifill threads.

PDRN (POLYDEOXYRIBONUCLEOTIDE) PCL (POLYCAPROLACTONE) THREADS

These threads are not yet registered in India. Available as cog threads with an 18-gauge cannula. Benefits of these threads are:

- Cell regeneration
- Collagen stimulation
- Enhances elasticity and longevity of results

NAMICA APTOS THREADS

Namica Aptos threads are the fourth generation threads with hyaluronic acid. The thread has shells of hyaluronic acid like droplets along the whole length of thread. The delivery of hyaluronic acid in tissue is controlled for prolonged release because of the capsules being of different sizes. The advantage of using these threads is superior improvement in skin quality compared to other PLCL [poly(L-lactide-Co-ε-caprolactone)] threads.[3]

CLINICAL PEARL

- Combining different threads even without the use of fillers can give a complete facelift if we tailor the threads according to different faces and areas of the face.

CONCLUSION

By understanding the characteristics and applications of different types of threads, practitioners can achieve natural, harmonious, and long lasting results while meeting individual needs of their patients. As thread technology continues to evolve, a combined use of different types of threads represents the future of thread based rejuvenation enabling more comprehensive and customized treatments.

REFERENCES

1. Hong GW, Hu H, Park SY, Wan J, Yi KH. What are the factors that enable thread lifting to last longer?. Cosmetics. 2024;11(2):42.
2. Hong GW, Kim SB, Park SY, Wan J, Yi KH. Thread Lifting Materials: A Review of Its Difference in Terms of Technical and Mechanical Perspective. Clinical, Cosmetic and Investigational Dermatology. 2024:999-1006.
3. Sulamanidze MA, Shiffman MA, Paikidze TG, Sulamanidze GM, Gavasheli LG. Facial lifting with APTOS threads. International Journal of Cosmetic Surgery and Aesthetic Dermatology. 2001;3(4):275-81.

CHAPTER 14

Dealing with Complications

Indu Ballani

INTRODUCTION

Threadlifts while minimally invasive and generally safe, are not entirely free from the risk of complications. As their popularity grows, so does the need for practitioners to be well equipped to handle potential adverse effects. This chapter focusses on recognizing, preventing and managing the complications of threadlifts.

BRUISING

This can happen with any injectable procedure. When cannulas are inserted in the right plane with minimal manipulation, the risk of bruising decreases **(Figs. 1A and B)**.[1] Needle may cause more bruising if it hits a blood vessel. Sometimes when bruising occurs in a deeper layer, it may present as yellowish discoloration after 4–5 days.

Management

Icing can be done immediately if a vessel is hit. Arnica or thrombophobe can be dabbed on the involved area. Anti-inflammatory may be needed if there is associated swelling. Settling down time may be 8–10 days.

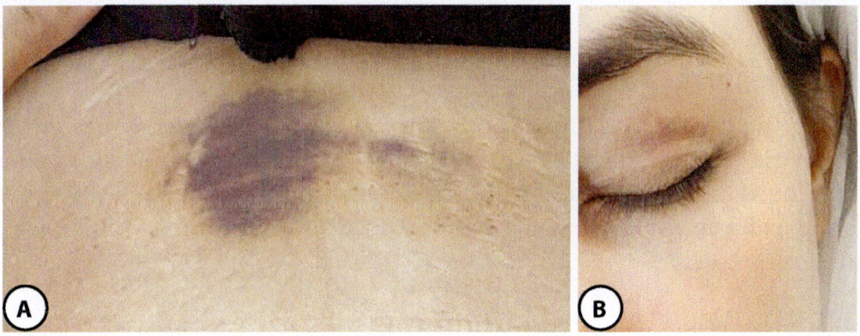

FIGS. 1A AND B: Bruise seen on the thread insertion site.

SWELLING AND INFLAMMATION

This is another complication which may occur with any injectable. Swelling is more when we use thicker threads and cannula and when there has been a lot of manipulation. This swelling may sometimes last for 3–4 weeks in case of cog threads.

Management

Anti-inflammatory tablets may be given regularly for 7–10 days.

DIMPLING AND IRREGULARITIES

This is a very common complication seen with cog threads. It happens due to superficial insertion of the cannula or the barbs giving traction on dermis, thus pulling it and causing dimpling.[1,2]

> **CLINICAL PEARL**
>
> While inserting the thread, if some dimpling becomes visible, withdraw the cannula by holding the projecting end of the thread against the cannula, so that the thread does not slide inside totally.

Management

Advance the cannula into the deeper layer and progress forward. After completing the procedure, try to massage and release the barbs, so that the dimpling is reduced. Usually dimpling reduces with the swelling in a week. In case the dimpling does not disappear even after a month, subcision can be done to release the barbs.

Radiofrequency (RF) sessions at weekly intervals can also help in reducing the dimpling.

ASYMMETRY

Asymmetry can occur due to pre-existing asymmetries, which look aggravated after the procedure or else if the vectors have not been marked symmetrically on both sides.

Management

Marking the vectors equally on both sides is very important. Noting previous asymmetries and pointing these to the patient before the procedure should always be done. Sometimes, major asymmetries may require extra material on one side or different entry points or vector direction to maintain the symmetry.

HEMATOMA

This may happen when a vessel is accidentally hit with needle threads or due to needle at entry point for cannula insertion.

Management includes icing, anti-inflammatory, and antibiotics. Steroids if needed can be prescribed.

INFECTION

This is an uncommon complication, which happens when proper aseptic measures have not been taken or when a hair enters an entry prick **(Fig. 2)**.[1-3]

Management

A short course of antibiotics is usually required to deal with the infection unless it is an atypical mycobacterial infection.

PROTRUSION, EXTRUSION, AND MIGRATION OF THREADS

Such a complication can occur if the thread barbs are weak or inserted in an area of animation (e.g., when marionette lines are crossed with threads).

Protrusion of the thread at entry point **(Figs. 3A and B)** can occur if the thread is not adequately pulled and tensioned before being cut close to the skin, to prevent this, it is essential to ensure that the thread is securely anchored and the excess is cut with precision. Additionally sliding the skin at entry point after cutting the thread ensures that the thread fully slides into the subcutaneous without entangling barbs in dermis. Sometimes in double needle threads, if the

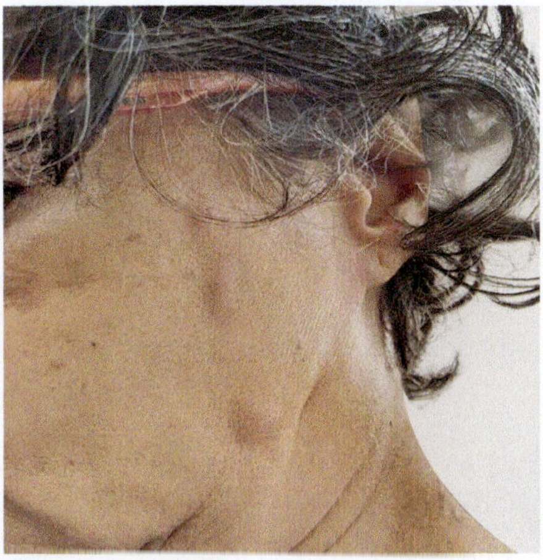

FIG. 2: Atypical mycobacterial infection after double needle threads.
Courtesy: Dr Lipi Gupta.

threads are fine and have not been cut properly at the exit point, there might be extrusion.

Management

The protruding thread can be pulled out and cut. If a nodule has formed at the exit point, due to protruding barb it can be subcised and the extra part of thread can be cut.

SIALOCELE

Parotid duct injury due to aggressive deep insertion may cause sialocele and parotid swelling **(Fig. 4)**.

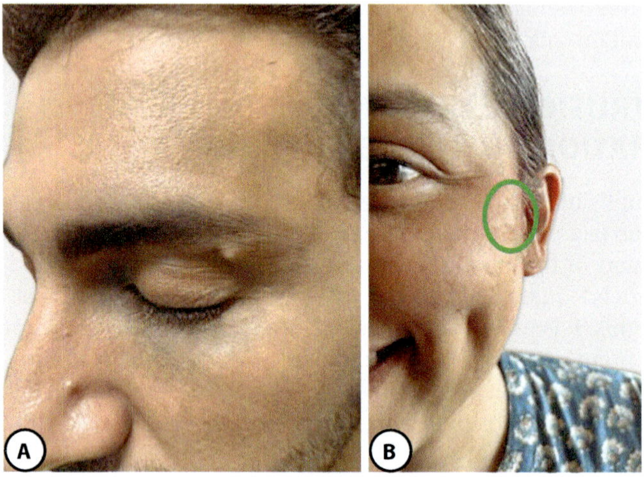

FIGS. 3A AND B: Nodule formation at the entry point.

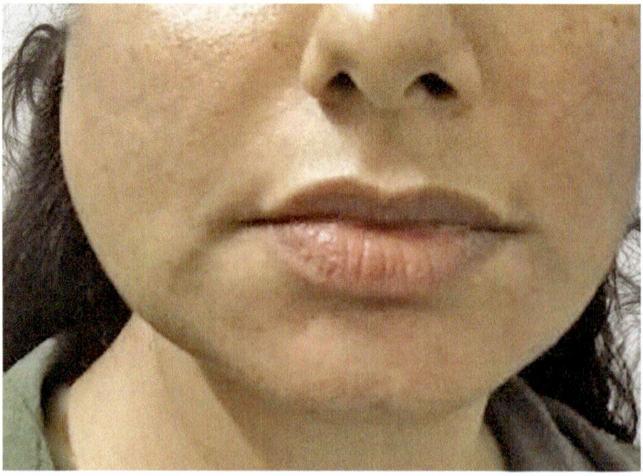

FIG. 4: Parotid swelling post thread insertion.

Management

Antibiotics may be required for 2–3 weeks. Botulinum toxin may be required in some cases.

CONCLUSION

Prevention remains the cornerstone of complication management, emphasizing the importance of proper patient selection, meticulous technique and adherence to postprocedure protocols.

Recognizing early warning signs,understanding underlying causes and implementing prompt and appropriate interventions are essential for optimal outcomes of our procedures.

REFERENCES

1. Bertossi D, Botti G, Gualdi A, Fundarò P, Nocini R, Pirayesh A, et al. Effectiveness, longevity, and complications of facelift by barbed suture insertion. Aesthet Surg J. 2019;39:241-7.
2. Wang CK. Complications of thread lift about skin dimpling and thread extrusion. Dermatol Ther. 2020;33(4):e13446.
3. Li YL, Li ZH, Chen XY, Xing WS, Hu JT. Facial Thread Lifting Complications in China: Analysis and Treatment. Plast Reconstr Surg Glob Open. 2021;9(9):e3820.

CHAPTER 15

Combination Procedures

Rashmi Sarkar, Damini Verma

INTRODUCTION

Facial aging is a gradual and complex process that affects everyone. As we age, changes in the soft tissue (fat and muscle) and bone of the face lead to loss of skin elasticity, decreased collagen production, sagging soft tissues, and appearance of jowls, nasolabial folds, and overall facial laxity. Although, traditional surgical facelifts offer effective results, but are invasive, costly, and require significant recovery time. Noninvasive and minimally invasive treatment modalities are gaining popularity due to their reduced downtime, elimination of need for general anesthesia, lower risk, and natural-looking outcomes.[1] Among these, thread lifting has emerged as a popular choice for facial rejuvenation. However, combining thread lifts with other treatment modalities will lead to more harmonious and more natural looking facial rejuvenation as effectively and as safely as possible. It will enhance both short-term and long-term outcomes, giving patients more comprehensive and sustained results.

This chapter will explore the synergy between thread lifts and other treatment modalities such as injectables, lasers, radiofrequency (RF), and energy-based devices in achieving a harmonious facial rejuvenation.

A BRIEF OVERVIEW OF THREAD LIFTS

Thread lifting is a minimally invasive procedure that has experienced a recent surge in popularity as interest in minimally invasive techniques for facial rejuvenation continues to grow. It carries several advantages over the traditional face lifts as it lifts the superficial musculoaponeurotic system (SMAS) to address facial ptosis by placing barbed sutures along the specific trajectories. It also stimulates collagen production in addition to providing an immediate lift that is characteristically seen in mid face and lower face. While thread lifts can offer impressive results, they are not a one-size-fits-all solution. Thread lifts can be combined with other modalities to address multiple signs of aging, such as volume loss, textural irregularities, pigmentation, and wrinkles and provide a more harmonious facial rejuvenation.[2]

COMBINATION TREATMENTS WITH THREAD LIFTS

Threads and Fillers

It is believed that with age, deep fat pads of face atrophies and superficial fat tend to reposition or hypertrophy. Along with this, there is also bony remodeling and weakening of supporting ligaments. It leads to volume loss, particularly in areas such as the cheeks, temples, and under the eyes and fat redistribution and protrusion that are mainly seen submentally in the jowl, lateral nasolabial fold, and lateral nasolabial crease. Dermal fillers, such as hyaluronic acid (HA) or calcium hydroxylapatite, restore lost volume by filling hollow areas and enhancing facial contours. When combined with thread lifts, dermal fillers can complement the lifting effect by volumizing specific areas that cannot be addressed by threads alone.

Protocol

Threads are typically done first to lift and reposition the skin, reducing jowls and facial sagging. After the threads are placed, fillers are injected to restore volume in areas such as the cheeks, lips, and tear troughs. There can be a gap of 2–3 weeks between these two modalities. They can also be done in same sessions in two different areas of face; e.g., fillers in mid-face and threads in lower face.

Threads and Botulinum Toxin

Repetitive muscle contractions lead to dynamic wrinkles, such as crow's feet, frown lines, and forehead wrinkles. While thread lifts can reposition sagging skin, they are not designed to address dynamic wrinkles. This is where botulinum toxin comes in as by temporarily paralyzing the muscles responsible for these lines, it reduces the appearance of wrinkles, offering a smoother skin surface.

Protocol

- Botulinum toxin can be administered before or 2 weeks after thread lifts. Botox relaxes the muscles responsible for dynamic wrinkles, complementing the lifting effect of the threads.
- If a treatment involves using fillers, botulinum toxin, and threads in the same session, then we must be careful of using one modality in one area of face. For example, toxins can be used on upper face, fillers in midface, and threads in lower face. If we are planning to do threads first, then fillers can be done after a gap of 3–4 weeks **(Flowchart 1)**.[3]
- A generalized rule for injectables can be "Never inject at the same time in the same area and same plane".

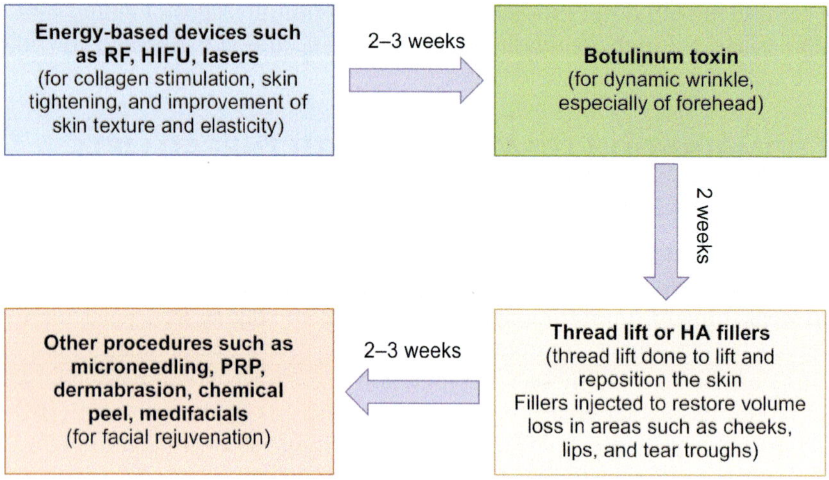

FLOWCHART 1: Flow of procedures for combination therapy for skin antiaging.
(HA: hyaluronic acid; HIFU: high-intensity focused ultrasound; PRP: platelet-rich plasma; RF: radiofrequency)

Threads and Radiofrequency

Radiofrequency treatment modalities, such as thermage, use energy to heat the deeper layers of the skin, stimulating collagen and elastin production. This results in skin tightening over time, improving skin texture and elasticity. Combining RF with thread lifts can enhance the lifting effect and prolong the longevity of the results by further tightening the skin and promoting collagen remodeling.[4]

Protocol

Radiofrequency should be done before to avoid unnecessary manipulation of the face when threads are placed as bruising or displacement of the products may occur if sequence is incorrect. Thread lift should be done after 2–3 weeks of RF therapy. RF should be avoided for at least 12–14 weeks after thread lift.

Threads and Laser Resurfacing

While thread lifts focus on lifting the underlying tissues, laser treatments such as fractional CO_2 or Erbium can address fine lines, hyperpigmentation, scars, and textural irregularities. Combining these two modalities allows for comprehensive facial rejuvenation, both at the skin's surface and deeper levels.

Protocol

Thread lift should be done after 2–3 weeks of completion of laser therapy. Laser should be avoided for at least 12–14 weeks after thread lift. Threads can be given in between sessions of laser hair reduction without any problem. After the threads, the next session should be scheduled after minimum 3 weeks.

Threads and Ultrasound

Ultrasound energy devices like high-intensity focused ultrasound (HIFU) targets the deep dermis and the SMAS to stimulate collagen production and tighten the skin. It offers skin tightening similar to thread lifts but focuses on gradual collagen stimulation. When combined with thread lifting, ultrasound can prolong the lift by enhancing collagen support.

Protocol

Similar to other resurfacing and rejuvenating procedures, thread lift should be done after 2–3 weeks of ultrasound therapy. HIFU should be avoided for at least 12–14 weeks after thread lift.[4]

Threads and Other Modalities such as Microneedling, Platelet-rich Plasma, Dermabrasion, Chemical Peel, and Medifacials

Microneedling creates microinjuries in the skin, promoting collagen production and allowing better penetration of topical treatments like platelet-rich plasma (PRP). PRP uses the patient's own platelets to stimulate healing and collagen synthesis. Dermabrasion and chemical peels lead to facial rejuvenation by reducing skin surface irregularities, photodamage, and pigmentation. Medifacials also deal with pigmentation, signs of aging, and photodamage. Combining these modalities with threads enhances the overall rejuvenation by addressing both lifting and skin quality.

Protocol

There should be a gap of 2–3 weeks between thread lifts and other facial rejuvenating procedures **(Flowchart 1)**.

When performing combination treatments, it is essential to consider the patient's unique anatomy, skin type, and aging pattern. Educating the patient about the realistic outcomes, risks, and benefits of the recommended procedures ensures they make informed decisions and undergo the safest and most effective treatments. Tailoring the treatment plan for each individual ensures that the modalities work synergistically for a natural, harmonious outcome. Proper scheduling of treatments is also critical to avoid overlapping side effects and ensure optimal results.

CONCLUSION

Thread lifting, when combined with other modalities, offers a comprehensive approach to facial rejuvenation. Multiple types of antiaging treatments are required to address the various etiologies of facial aging. To enhance results, thread lifts can be combined with other treatments such as injectable fillers and neurotoxins, which help to restore facial volume and smooth fine lines. These treatments can also be complemented by laser resurfacing or chemical peels to address issues within the epidermis and superficial dermis. By utilizing a combination of these modalities, both clinicians and patients can benefit from the synergistic effects, addressing the various aspects of facial aging more comprehensively.

CLINICAL PEARL

Multiple antiaging treatment modalities such as fillers and neurotoxins can be combined with thread lift, as it offers a comprehensive approach to facial rejuvenation. They can also be done in same sessions in two different areas of face; e.g., botulinum in upper face, fillers in mid-face, and threads in lower face. It can be further combined with energy-based devices, laser resurfacing, or chemical peels to address facial aging more comprehensively.

REFERENCES

1. Beer KR. Combined treatment for skin rejuvenation and soft-tissue augmentation of the aging face. J Drugs Dermatol. 2011;10(2):125-32.
2. Tong LX, Rieder EA. Thread-Lifts: A Double-Edged Suture? A Comprehensive Review of the Literature. Dermatol Surg. 2019;45(7):931-40.
3. Moon H, Fundaro SP, Goh CL, Hau KC, Paz-Lao P, Salti G. A review on the combined use of soft tissue filler, suspension threads, and botulinum toxin for facial rejuvenation. J Cutan Aesth Surg. 2021;14(2):147-55.
4. Fabi S, Pavicic T, Braz A, Green JB, Seo K, van Loghem JA. Combined aesthetic interventions for prevention of facial ageing, and restoration and beautification of face and body. Clin Cosmet Investig Dermatol. 2017;10:423-9.

CHAPTER 16

My Learnings from Korea

Indu Ballani

In this chapter, I will enlist my experience of learning advanced techniques from the renowned Dr Kim Wooran[1] in Korea. Dr Kim is a pioneer in the field of nonsurgical facial rejuvenation, particularly through the use of cog threads for contouring the face. A session with Dr Kim provided me with a deeper understanding of the vectors for thread insertion and use of different types of threads according to target area.

1. Patient was under intravenous (IV) sedation anesthesia for the whole procedure with proper monitoring.
2. 18–20 threads were inserted on each side for full face.
3. Instead of putting two threads from one point of entry Dr Kim inserted them from two different points to pull up an area.
4. Used Foxy Flex threads for cheeks with curved cannula according to shape of the cheeks **(Fig. 1)**.

---

[1]Dr Kim is a representative director of Wayne Plastic Surgery, who considers and strives for the entire process, including naturalness, safety, and postsurgical care.

- Adjunct Professor, Asan Medical Center, Seoul
- Seoul Asan Medical Center Specialist/Resident/Trainee
- Alumni of Asan Plastic Surgery Department in Seoul
- Completion of the highest level medical management course at Seoul National University College of Medicine
- Korea University Graduate School of Business Administration (MBA)
- Former Director of The Plastic Surgery Apgujeong Branch
- Former Director of Thewell Plastic Surgery Bundang Branch
- Member of IPRAS International Society of Plastic Surgery
- Member of Oculoplastic Research Group, Korean Society of Plastic Surgery
- Member of Rhinoplasty Research Group, Korean Society of Plastic Surgery
- Member of Facial Contour Research Group, Korean Society of Plastic Surgery
- Member of the Local Plastic Surgery Research Group of the Korean Society of Plastic Surgery
- Member of Micro-Invasion Research Group, Korean Society of Plastic Surgery

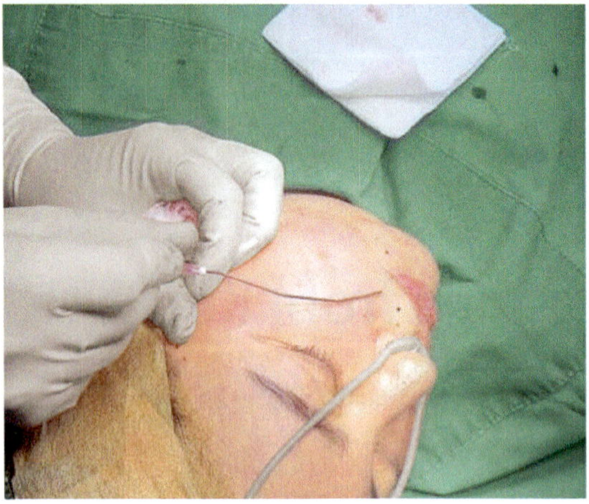

FIG. 1: Foxy Flex threads.

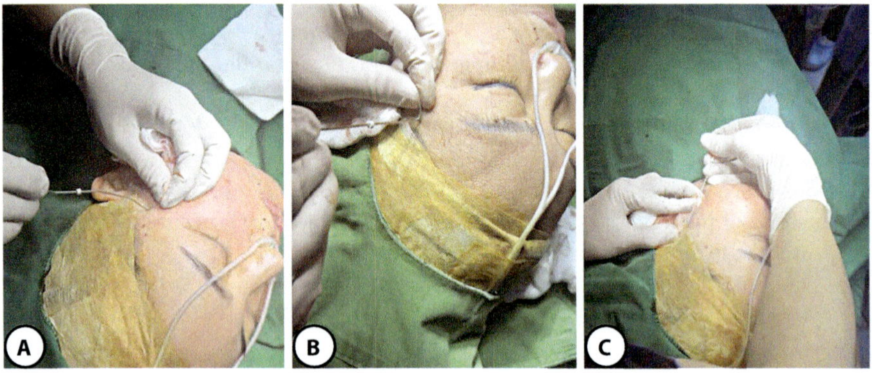

FIGS. 2A TO C: Taking out the cannula and reinserting the thread upward into the temple.

5. The cog threads were reinserted upward in a different direction to improve the pull of threads and avoid wasting any thread **(Figs. 2A to C)**.
   Eyebrow threads: Three threads were inserted on each side from three separate points, one of the points being on medial side which we are afraid to do due to supraorbital vessels.
6. Special fixing type of threads (SE fixing type) were inserted from the jawline to temple to improve the lifting effect **(Fig. 3)**.

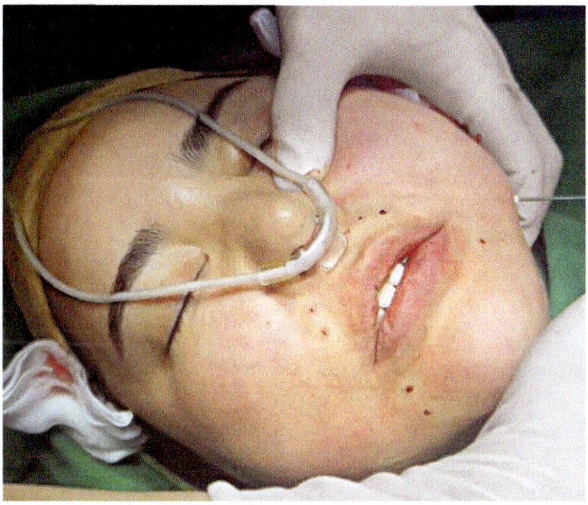

FIG. 3: SE fixing type threads inserted in a reverse direction.

CLINICAL PEARL

- Reverse vectors on the cheek along with Foxy Flex threads along the nasolabial fold (NLF) vector give best results for lifting the NLF.

Index

Page numbers followed by *f* refer to figure, *fc* refer to flowchart and *t* refer to table.

O

P

R

S

T